Don't Just Give Me

That
Old Time Religion

Don't Just Give Me

That Old Time Religion

Religion and Mental Well-being among African American Women

Christine Y. Wiley

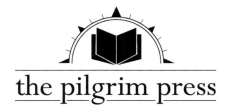

the pilgrim press

The Pilgrim Press, 1300 East 9th Street
Cleveland, Ohio 44114
thepilgrimpress.com

Published 2025.

Library of Congress Cataloging-in-Publication Data on file.
LCCN: 2024949585

ISBN 978-0-8298-0065-4 (paper)
ISBN 978-0-8298-0068-5 (ebook)

Printed in The United States of America on acid-free paper.

Contents

Preface

I had an entirely different idea for the topic for my doctoral dissertation that this book is based on. When I entered my doctoral program, I thought my research would address the attitudes of African Americans towards the LGBTQ community. The church I co-pastored with my husband was a Black inner-city church that became open and affirming of LGBTQ people in 2004. A storm brewed when my husband and I performed two Holy Union ceremonies of a gay and a lesbian couple in 2007.

As I moved through my studies, I realized that I had become somewhat annoyed with part of the Black Church that not only shut out the LGBTQ community but also limited the role of Black women with its theology and traditions. Teaching practical courses in seminary and experiencing students who were products of their conservative churches was what propelled me to do further study in the first place. I was already a licensed professional counselor, having gotten a doctor of ministry degree in pastoral psychotherapy some years earlier. But now, the field of social work attracted me. The preamble to the code of ethics of the national Association of Social Workers states: "The primary mission of the social work profession is to enhance human well-being and help meet the basic human needs of all people, with particular attention to the needs and empowerment of people who are vulnerable, oppressed, and living in poverty." Having developed a sense of well-being and feeling empowered as a woman who is religious and who has had experiences with sexism, racism, and even trauma had me curious about other Black women and how they negotiated their everyday lives.

I reflected on what it was like for me to be the only Baptist woman student in my divinity school at that time in the early 1980s and some of the subtle and not so subtle discrimination I experienced. I thought about what it was like for me to be the first woman to be licensed to preach, and later ordained at my church. I experienced some of the internalized oppression of women in the church as some said, "I just want to hear a man's voice." I also experienced the sweetness of deeper spirituality both in my church and in my seminary.

I sat with women in my counseling office, some in tears, some with overwhelming anger, and some who just relinquished themselves, who were told by their pastors that if they just did what their husbands told them to do then everything would be alright. I counseled women who had insurmountable stress as they had the responsibility of raising a family and were the head of their household with meager income. Often, I had to be case manager, counselor, and pastor.

As I reflect, I think about my mother. She was a British-born Black woman who married an American Black man in the military in the 1950s and came to the United States with two children and pregnant with my brother. This was a strange and new place for her, but her wisdom and motherly wit nourished her five children. I think about my sister, Lorraine, who came after me. She adopted two children and died of asthma at a young age with all the stress and pressure she went through as a single mom. I think of my sister Theresa, who lost her only son. He was only twenty-one. He had an embolism in his leg that traveled to his heart and killed him. She covers her grief, but as she sits with my children and grandchildren it is still palpable. I think of my eldest daughter Aiyana, who is a therapist and has done her own work and helps other Black women who also love God. I think of my youngest daughter Samira, who came out to us at the age of twenty-one while a student at The Juilliard School. Now she is negotiating this world as a Black gay woman with a wife and a young daughter. I also think of my son Joshua, and my husband Dennis, men who treat women with respect, kindness, and care.

Finally, I think of the women in this study who did not know me but trusted me and shared their stories of pain, joy, spirituality, ambivalence, and resilience. Despite a sometimes-rocky road, I am so grateful to my Lord and Savior Jesus Christ, who through this process helped me to believe in the Black Church again and called me to this work. To all these women and others like them, I am so grateful that I have become acquainted with them and the ways they have negotiated religion and life while striving for a positive sense of mental well-being.

One

Finding New Wineskins: Herstory

Give me that old-time religion, give me that old-time religion.
Give me that old time religion, it's good enough for me!
It's good enough for our mothers, it's good enough for our mothers.
It's good enough for our mothers, it's good enough for me.

I remember singing this song in church. There is something about it that runs deep in Black Church tradition and brings a smile to people's faces. Religion and the church have been good for many, particularly African Americans; however, there is also something else about "that old time religion" that can be stifling and oppressive. Some speak of being hurt by religion. I think of days in the past when young teen girls became pregnant and were put out of the church. Gay people had to hide in the church to escape shame and ostracizing, which is still true today in many cases. Women, who outnumbered men and raised most of the money, were not allowed to have significant leadership in the church.

The African American Heritage Hymnal preludes this hymn with a scripture: "I am reminded of your sincere faith . . . first in your grandmother . . . and your mother . . . and now, I am sure, lives in you" (2 Timothy 1:5). We may have gotten some of the first tenets of our faith from our mothers and grandmothers, but our experience of religion and the transformation that happens within us as we reflect on our lives and what we have been taught may require us to "eat the meat and spit out the bones." My own experience of religion is one in which my mind, heart, and understanding have been transformed as I pay attention to the scripture: "Do not conform to the pattern of this world but be transformed by the renewing of your mind" (Romans 12:2 NIV). This means to "think differently" as one reflects on their experience with God, scripture, spirituality, and religion. As an African American clergy woman, and a scholar in the field of social work, my experience, study, and theological reflection have had me thinking differently than what has been presented in religious tradition throughout my life.

My life started as a child in a military family. My father was stationed at March Air Force Base, California where I remember going to the Protestant Chapel for worship and to Sunday school, which was held at the elementary school I attended. These two buildings were walking distance from one another, so I could leave Sunday school and walk over to the chapel for worship. Going to worship was such a joy for me. I remember literally skipping and smiling as I went from Sunday school to the chapel. During this time in the 1950s and early 1960s, there weren't that many African Americans in the Air Force, so often my mother, who sang in the choir, and I, who always sat in the front row of the chapel, were the only African Americans in the service. From when I was about five years old until we were transferred to Germany at the age of twelve, I never really noticed being "a fly in the milk" in this environment. During my time in worship, I loved singing the hymns and even listening to the preacher. In my early years, I had never heard a Black preacher, and most of the chaplains at that time were White and came out of the Lutheran and Episcopal or Methodist traditions. I remember one Sunday a White chaplain from the South came to preach and I was so excited. He could really preach! The rise and fall of his voice and the simple words he used helped me to lean in and pay even more attention than usual.

The attention to my Black Church experience also points to my own history as a Black woman. My mother was a British born Black woman. My father, a Black man raised in Mississippi, was a non-commissioned officer in the Air Force. He married my mother when he was stationed in England. My mother had no aversion to White people because her mother was White and many of her friends and neighbors where she grew up were White. She was a first generation British-born Black woman, where fathers were from the Caribbean or Africa and the mothers were British and White. My mother felt comfortable with White people, so she had no difficulty in the base housing environment, where there were very few people of color, at the California Air Force Base in the 1950s and 1960s. This was at the height of segregation in our country.

Differences between Black and White people became more apparent, and my eyes were clearly opened when our family went on vacation, driving from Riverside, California, to Hattiesburg, Mississippi, my father's place of birth and home. We had to sleep at rest stops along the way. My father was the only driver and there were no hotels we could stay in at that time due to Jim Crow laws. While once traveling through Texas, we used The Negro Travelers Green Book. When a big storm started brewing, we were guided to a private home where our family of two parents and four children could stay for the night. It took us five days to get to Mississippi from California and five days to get back. When we arrived in Hattiesburg, I had not seen so many Black people in one place in my entire short life! My grandmother had thirteen children, two of whom died. All her boys went to college and the girls all went to some kind of trade school. My father had gone to Morehouse College, and one of my uncles went to graduate school at Harvard. There were stories of civil rights leaders who had come to stay at my grandmother's home. Her family had donated the land on which the church, Morning Star Baptist Church, stood and all the family belonged to. I remember picking up a comic book that was all about the Rev. Dr. Martin Luther King, Jr. When I saw the cover, I asked my grandmother who he was. Mama Jones as we called her said, "Chile, you never heard of Rev. Dr. Martin Luther King? Your parents never told you about him? Read that book." I was truly getting a new education about what it meant to be a Black person in this country. I read that comic book and started to see myself and my place in American society differently.

The experience I will never forget about Hattiesburg is going to church on Sunday. First, we would have quite a breakfast of bacon and eggs, pork chops, grits, and biscuits. We would then go to Sunday school, and afterwards we would go to worship, which seemed to last almost all day. We would come home and eat another meal of fried chicken, greens, sweet potatoes, and okra. After this it was time for Baptist Training Union. I really did not understand the purpose of BTU, but they were teaching us how to pray in public. Then some- times after BTU, we would go back to evening service. On Sunday, you spent the entire day in church. In Sunday school, the children asked my siblings and me questions like, "Why do you talk so proper like White folks? Do you go to school with little White children?" They could hardly believe it when we said we went to Sunday school and church with White people. The most exhilarating time for me was the Sunday morning worship. It was hot, but the overhead fans made it cooler. Even though it was hot, the men wore ties and short sleeve shirts on these days, and the women wore their best dresses. We as children also wore our best. The girls had to make sure we had lotion on our legs and wore our black patent leather shoes that were always so shiny. There were no musical instruments. An older man would come in front of the congregation and chant a line of a hymn to the congregation. In response, the congregation would then draw out that line and sing together in unison without any musical instruments. The words were familiar, but the melody was different. The voices would float and slide. I learned about common meter hymns and short meter. Sister Matt was an older woman who walked with a cane. When the congregation was singing, she would drop her cane to the beat on the wooden floor. It was something to hear and behold. I had not experienced this in the Protestant Chapel! I learned that this metered hymn went back to the days of slavery in the African American tradition.

But then came the preacher. I had never experienced preaching that was so intoxicating. First of all, it did not seem that the preacher used any notes or manuscript, and he was very demonstrative in his delivery of the sermon. This celebratory style of preaching impacted my mind and intellect even as a young person, but it also appealed to my emotions. Towards the end of the sermon, the preacher chanted the sermon. There was a melody and call and response where the congregation spoke back to the preacher. We not only heard the sermon, but we felt the sermon. I learned later that this was called whooping.

Those experiences of Hattiesburg stayed in the back recesses of my mind. As I got a little older in California, I remember looking at the television and seeing police beating Black people in Alabama and siccing dogs on them. I remember thinking, "If I were there, they would do that to me." My desire to do something to help my people was kindled in my heart.

Over the years, after working in mental health nursing, attending seminary, serving in a social justice-oriented church as a minister and pastor, and getting a doctor of ministry degree in pastoral psychotherapy at Garrett Seminary, and a doctor of philosophy in social work at Howard University School of Social Work, my concern for justice and alleviating those who are oppressed became deeply embedded within me. The School of Social Work has a core value called The Black Perspective: "It reaffirms the richness, productivity and vigor of the lives of African Americans, Africans, people of color and marginalized and oppressed people in other parts of the world and emphasizes the delineation of ways in which the strengths of African Americans can be used to respond to oppressive and discriminatory systems." I have internalized this perspective as I work with Black people who have experienced disparagement and abuse in our society, but have had the resilience to work through the difficulties and succeed.

An understanding of the relationship that African American women have with religion today requires looking at the religious components that follow African ancestry even before the atrocities of the Atlantic slave trade. Cook and Wiley have stated that, "As people of African descent, African Americans have inherited a cultural legacy that perceives spirituality as a foundation of personal and communal life." According to the late John Mbiti, in traditional African culture there is no separation of spirituality and religion. Everything that the African is involved in or does is a part of their lived spirituality. This is true whether it is the individual or the community. The understanding is that if you are human, then you are in community, and if you are in community, then you have a relationship with God. This understanding frames Africans' educational and cultural ways of being. It also infuses their occupations, political alignments, and their economic enterprises. Religion is mixed into people's lives. They live and breathe religion; it is not pigeon-holed into religious philosophy or code of belief. God is seen in everyone and everything. This God is seen as the Almighty, the creator, the Alpha and Omega. A South African phrase called Ubuntu means "I am because we are and because we are, therefore, I am." Because African spirituality and religion are communal, caring for one another and paying attention to the joys and sufferings of the community as a whole and as individuals are integral to it. Those who have died are seen as spirit ancestors who are still active in people's lives to help them.

Mbiti indicated that God is seen as the creator of the universe and all things. This God is all powerful, all merciful, a just God, a holy and all-knowing God who is omnipresent, never changing, and limitless. In some African traditions, God is seen as father; in others, mother; and in others, as friend. Some also believe that God has created a number of sky and earth spirits that explain the mysteries surrounding them.

As Africans were stolen from the motherland and brought to this country as slaves, slaveholders tried to destroy their religion and beliefs. But these new African Americans found strength in their traditions under the brutality of slavery. They would meet under cover and find strength in the music, songs, and dance from Africa. Drums were played and fortitude was gained as they received and became united with the Spirit. This was a time of healing, and these African Americans were able to feel renewed power and vitality.

It was not long before the European church tried to present Christ to slaves to "save souls." Slave holders did not like this because of political, social, and economic reasons. The authors Lincoln and Mamiya felt that the slave holders did not want their slaves thinking that all were equal under the cross. However, slave holders' perspective changed; they used the religion to make sure their slaves were obedient and docile. These resilient African American slaves took a different view of Christianity. They adapted their own African sense of spirituality and religion to Christianity, especially those components that brought them consolation and relief in the midst of the abuses of slavery. They would meet in the hush harbors, a place often in the bushes away from the plantation or house where they could meet in secret to testify, sing songs, and pray. They adapted their own African traditional religion within Christianity. The slave masters emphasized "Slaves, obey your earthly masters with respect and fear, and with sincerity of heart, just as you would obey Christ" (Ephesians 6:5, NIV). The African American slaves, however, saw Jesus as a liberator. They identified with the torture and persecution of Jesus. They were strengthened by the determination and endurance of Jesus, and they found power and hope in his resurrection.

In the late 1800s, due to overt racism in the White church where African Americans had to sit in the balcony and undergo other abuses, independent African American churches were formed that were controlled by African Americans. These independent churches had freedom to bring forth their own spiritual style and interpretation. The churches had an understanding that they were children of God instead of seeing themselves as three-fifths human as noted in the US Constitution. This sense of freedom was what led these churches to fight for equality during the civil rights movement.

Pastors and church members, activists and lay workers organized a movement for liberation from Jim Crow, racism, and an unequal justice system. Pastors used their pulpits to speak to the issue of justice and equality for Black people. Churches provided financial support for the movement. They preached about internalized oppression so that African Americans would know that they were equal to any white people, that they were "a royal priesthood, a holy nation, God's special possession" (1 Peter 2:9, NIV). These Black people could love their brown skin of so many hues and love their African heritage and be proud of themselves. Black men and women found comfort in the Black Church.

Black women have not had an easy time in the church or the world at large, even though religion and church have been prominent in their lives. They have used their faith and spirituality to propel them to action amid oppression both within and outside of the church. Women's mission organizations in the church were designed to support the individual churches and their denominations. The women learned administrative abilities and learned to work together and value themselves and their proficiencies. These organizations positioned women to become aware of their stature in the church and brought forth the beginnings of Black feminist awareness. Black women had a significant place and purpose in religion and in the church. Historically, Black women have been called the "backbone of the Black Church."

Some of these mission organizations became so strong that they had more power than the churches they represented, which was a response to discrimination by men in the church. Social activism became primary as Black women understood that their Christian mission was addressing sexism within the church and racism in all its facets. Combating classism was also an issue. Some women, such as Nannie Helen Burroughs, advocated for diverse leadership of women regardless of class, noting that working class women have as much right to be in leadership as Black women of privilege. We have heard of the names of early Black women activists such as Sojourner Truth, Harriet Tubman, Mary Church Terrell, Ida B. Wells, and Mary McLeod Bethune. Much work was done by Black church women whose organizations also established Black settlement houses in several cities to address issues related to poverty.

Although women were not always in the forefront during the civil rights movement, they were the ones doing the organizing to keep the movement going. Working in this movement was seen as essential to the religious lives of these women. We have heard and seen the works of Fannie Lou Hamer, Rosa Parks, and Coretta Scott King, but it is important for us to understand that there were many Black women who were in the trenches during the civil rights movement. Many of these women have become invisible as historians and others have focused on Black religious organizations and influential Black male ministers. It is only recently that works of research on Black women's civil rights activism has started to emerge in significant numbers. Countless Black women from the end of slavery until now have seen it as part of their religious responsibility to pursue racial uplift and social liberation as a duty to God. During the civil rights movement, Black churches had to organize and galvanize, participating in rallies and marches and suffering violence from police, being sprayed by fire hoses, and being bitten by attack dogs. There have been many parts of the Black Church that have stood up against oppression and blatant attacks on the Black community.

At the same time, many Black churches did not want to be involved and "stir up" difficulty with the White community.

Just as during the civil rights era, our country has today heavily shifted towards right-wing ideology. After President Donald Trump's defeat in the 2020 presidential election, he encouraged a mob of his supporters to attack the United States Capitol building in Washington, DC. It is clear that Trump incited the attack. Militia groups such as the Proud Boys and the Oath Keepers, along with the QAnon movement, have been clear about their white supremacist ideology, and many of their members have been charged with seditious conspiracy and been imprisoned. Two historic Black churches in Washington, DC had their "Black Lives Matter" signs on their buildings burned and destroyed during a pro-Trump rally. The churches were the Asbury United Methodist church, founded in 1936, and Metropolitan African Methodist Episcopal Church, where Frederick Douglas's funeral was held in 1895. Threatening messages were also left by the Proud Boys on the churches' voice mail. These acts of racial terror and religious violence, as stated by Yolanda Pierce, former Dean of the Howard University School of Divinity, illustrated the continued racism and violence towards Blacks in our country. The Metropolitan African Methodist Episcopal Church sued the Proud Boys and received a one-million-dollar settlement. This violence is reminiscent of the threats and violence faced by Black people and Black churches in the 1800s from groups such as the Ku Klux Klan.

I remember the 2017 Women's March, a significant protest the day after the inauguration of Donald Trump as the US president. The protest was sparked by Trump's policy stances and language, which were viewed as sexist and posed a danger to women's rights. On a Sunday morning, there were about ten white male protestors who stormed into my Black Church, Covenant Baptist United Church of Christ, carrying signs against LGBTQ rights that said "Faggots are going to hell," and yelling that we as a congregation were going to hell. They also had signs against abortion. Perhaps they were aware that earlier my husband, Rev. Dr. Dennis Wiley, and I led a delegation of clergy to bless a new Planned Parenthood facility in Washington, DC. They had bull horns and disrupted our Sunday school. My church is an Open and Affirming Church for LGBTQ people and all people, and we have a history of speaking truth to power. The men and women of our church escorted the protestors out of the church by gently holding their arms. The women as well as the men felt just as empowered to act and not only speak truth to power, but to act. As the pastor of the church, I called the police. The protestors, after having been escorted out of the church, were on the sidewalk shouting into their bull horns and blocking parishioners from coming into the church. The police told me they had a right to protest. When I called the commander to ask that they move across the street, he said it was up to the officer in charge and he would not have the police move the protestors to the other side of the street. It was only when I was in the Mayors Faith Leaders meeting that I was told this should not have happened, but it was too late by then. The action that morning by men and women of our church and the action of its pastors in leading a blessing at the planned Parenthood Clinic illustrate how the spirituality and the prophetic understanding of daring to speak for and act on God's direction can show up, and how religion can intervene into culture, politics, race, and gender.

Religion has been a beneficial tool for my own life. There are times in my life, as a Black woman, wife, daughter, friend, social worker, educator, and pastor, that religion and spirituality have allowed me to ground myself in an identity that aids my own sense of self and gives me direction on how to navigate those roles. I think about when I was a young married woman with an infant and my first husband left me and my infant daughter. I remember being so sad for so long and even though I was a clinician, I was not able to see the forest for the trees and realize that I was depressed. When I got to a place of despair, my coping mechanism was prayer, crying out to God to help me. Going to worship held me up as I felt the Spirit of God. I remember crying cleansing tears when the pastor's sermon spoke to my condition. Reading scripture helped to put my life in perspective. It was my religion and spirituality that got me to a place of healing and wholeness. As I look back on that time, I am amazed at how I see God's movement in my life. I have since remarried and have three wonderful children and six amazing grandchildren. I also think about how my many roles of wife, mother, pastor, and therapist could also be overwhelming. I had become a "human-doing," moving from one role to the other and often not having a chance to breathe. I realized that religion by itself was not enough. This was a time when I decided to go into therapy. I learned that I had taken on this role of super woman which so many Black women take on, taking care of everyone except themselves. It was in that sacred space of sitting with my therapist that I realized I was ok. I didn't need to prove myself to anyone. I was already worthy, and I could give myself permission to take care of myself. I realized that yes, my religion and spirituality were important and helpful, but also intentionally addressing my mental health was critical.

I often think about how, when sitting in the counseling room as a therapist, somewhere in the mix of our meeting I get a good history of my client. Amid my questions, I may ask them if spirituality has a place in their lives. Invariably, they share with me their experience in the church. Some will also talk about how prayer has been helpful for them. I wonder whether professionals who work with Black women really understand their plight. Black women experience discrimination and marginalization at a higher rate than any other group. Black women try to live as whole human beings as they deal with and negotiate historical trauma, their experience of racism, sexism, and classism, and discrimination based on socioeconomic status, education, and mental health. They use their spirituality and religion to help them while they traverse the realities of their day-to-day lives.

It is important to understand that religion and religious activities have served as coping mechanisms for individuals, and religion is one of the core African American cultural values. Based on this insight, it is possible to see how mental well-being and participation in religious activities connect in the lives of African American women. Although spirituality is different from religion, religious involvement and religious institutions can be gateways to deeper spirituality.

Black women are the most religious people in the United States. Religion can point one to spirituality, and faith communities have served as a principal place in which Black women are able to discuss and interact regarding the trials of being both Black and a woman in a racist and sexist society. As culture has shifted over time, other ideologies have been interwoven into the African American religious experience. In addition to the traditional concern for community, women have now come to see that spirituality includes caring for their own well-being. They see the need to promote health and spirituality such as taking care of one's body, mind, and spirit. It is common knowledge that health disparities are rampant in the Black community. Self-care is not only spiritual and religious, but also biblical. First Corinthians 6:19–20 states, "Do you not know that your bodies are temples of the Holy Spirit, who is in you, whom you have received from God? You are not your own; you were bought with a price. Therefore, honor God with your bodies." Taking care of oneself includes paying attention to the body, what you put into your body, and how you exercise and take care of your body. It also means recognizing oneself as a spiritual being and nurturing this part of yourself. Another important area is one's mental health. All the stressors and even trauma that Black women endure can lead to difficulty with mental health.

Today there are more congregations paying attention to the whole person. This includes not only having health ministries dedicated to physical health including nutrition, exercise classes, blood pressure monitoring, diabetes screening, and cancer education. Many churches also now have counseling centers with licensed therapists offering individual, couples, and family therapy along with a myriad of support groups. This is not just a characteristic of the mega church—many smaller congregations are also trying to address the issues of health and wholeness. Pastors are getting more training and are networking with outside groups and agencies to bring services to their communities to address physical health and mental health for their parishioners and the community.

The ability to use religious resources during stress, difficulty, or everyday life can be seen as coping mechanisms that impact positive mental well-being and health. Within the community, Black religious institutions have served as a nucleus for African Americans, and particularly Black women. It is imperative for those working with Black women to understand the centrality of spirituality and faith. Although not all Black women are members of organized religion, mental health providers, social workers, and community providers need to understand the strengths and coping skills of Black women and be perceptive to the part that religion and spirituality might play. Sometimes Black women are stereotyped and judged regarding their involvement in religious activities or questioned about their spiritual beliefs. Providers must be intent on listening to and understanding how viewpoints on religion or spirituality influence women.

In a survey conducted among therapists who were members of the Association for Behavioral and Cognitive Therapies, approximately half of the sample reported a strong sense of spirituality. However, religious affiliation, belief in God, religious practice, and intrinsic religiosity were substantially lower than that of the general population of the United States. In addition, thirty-six percent reported discomfort in addressing issues of spirituality and religion; nineteen percent reported never inquiring about religion or spirituality; and seventy-one percent reported little-to-no previous training in this area. Today, more therapists are addressing religion and spirituality in their practices. A Washington Post article acknowledges that Americans' mental health is at the lowest point in history. There are a growing number of clinicians who believe that religion and spirituality have tools that can help with today's mental health crisis. Even though religion and spirituality are often not addressed in educational programs that train clinicians, therapists working with Black women must not be shy in assessing where women are in their involvement in religion. With the permission of women, using spiritual techniques can be remarkably helpful when persons are wrestling with deep existential questions. Black women may ask questions such as "God, why is this happening to me? What is the meaning and purpose of my life?" This is indicative of a spiritual problem, not a psychological problem. We know that deep trouble in a person's life can affect them physically, emotionally, and psychologically, which can lead to their health deteriorating. The Post article states that spiritual distress can increase the incidence of heart disease and other disorders as well as depression, anxiety, and thoughts of suicide.

In my own practice of psychotherapy, I will sometimes ask Black women clients who are under quite a bit of stress: "What has helped you in the past?" Often, they will tell me they have called on God, or they have prayed. We then talk about how this has worked for them, which sometimes moves towards a discussion of who this God is for them and whether they really trust God. I may find out that their God is a neglectful God or a punishing, God which can be a reflection of a parent's behavior or some other significant person in their lives. In our work together, they can finally get to a realization that they have not held a true sense of who God is and start to move towards developing a more holistic view of a loving God that they are able to have a real relationship with. Recognizing how important spirituality is for Black women can help organizations that fund positive programs and the faith community to work together to provide support and solutions for issues specific to Black women.

For a number of years in multiple seminaries, I taught practical theology courses such as field studies, church administration, and pastoral counseling. It became concerning to me that so many students, particularly those coming out of the Black Church tradition, were so conservative in how they saw and negotiated the world. Many came out of denominations or churches that were exclusive in terms of who could become part of their church and not be designated a sinner. Some churches and/or denominations did not believe in the ordination of women; most did not have an open attitude toward the LGBTQQ community, nor were they open to reproductive rights for women, particularly abortion, even though women of color were the most affected by restrictions on abortion.

As I contemplated the empowerment of Black women and paid attention to the plight of Black people in this nation and the oppression of same gender loving folks, particularly in the Black community, I became very concerned with the mindset of these students. I had counseled many Black families, individuals, and particularly women. Women were overwhelmed with responsibilities, and many lived with addictions. Some were victims of domestic violence and had responsibility for children. I thought about myself and what propelled me to pursue religion and spirituality when I was feeling so low and depressed. How was I able to get to the place of positive mental well-being, and what did that look like? I know that religion for me meant attending church and using religious resources such as prayer, worship, and reading my bible. This allowed me to go deeper in my spirituality and had me contemplating the meaning and purpose of my life. As I worked with those who had experienced trauma and mental unrest in their lives, I became aware that I could be present with people as they shared their pain. Some of their pain had to do with overt racism they experienced in their lives. I had experienced racism in my life and understood where they were in their pain and anger.

Black women in these United States of America experience outright racism in their lives as well as microaggressions in their places of employment, the marketplace, and their communities. Those subtle penetrating but offensive comments or actions can be intentional or unintentional because racism is so deeply systemic in our society. Women also experience not only negative attitudes and behavior but overt patriarchal attitudes and treatment which put them into sexist gender roles. They are often devalued or discriminated against just because they are Black women. When the intersections of race and gender come together the injustices multiply, and the influence and capabilities of women can be stifled.

After teaching in theological schools for many years and counseling students who were students in a master of divinity program, I became aware of some of the inconsistencies between what religion said and what leaders, especially male leaders in the church, were actually doing. The religious conservatism of the church appeared to place women in boxes that were difficult for them to navigate. Only a small percentage of Black women clergy are senior pastors. Acknowledgement of both men and women in the church who are LGBTQ is also lacking in many places.

Weary of the views of men and women in the seminary and the church, I left teaching in the seminary to pursue an additional doctoral degree in social work. My passion for justice and healing of people took me in this direction. I soon found that many of these professors and soon-to-be policy makers, clinicians, researchers, and social activists went to the same Black churches and held some of the same ideology and theology that I was suspicious of. This is when I decided to explore what Black women really thought about religion. Did it help them? What did they think about it? Was there any part of it that was not helpful for them? The result of my research is the topic of this book.

Much research has been conducted on how religion is seen today among Black people. In the last four decades, an increasing volume of scientific work has appeared in the area of spirituality and religion of African Americans. A multidimensional extensive study by the federal Office of Minority Health explored the religious life of African American women from all walks of life to analyze how religion intersected and connected with their mental well-being in their day-to-day experience. Compared to other ethnicities of both genders, African American women are the most religious group in the United States, and spirituality and religion are known to help them in their life, benefitting their psychological well-being. A thorough study of African American women's religious involvement and understanding can help us to understand how religion can be a bridge to one's mental well-being.

My experiences with various religious, spiritual, and mental health spaces and my conversations with other Black women exploring these same areas have led me to pose three questions:

* How do African American women describe mental well-being?

* How do African American women perceive the role that religion plays in their lives?

* How does religion make African American women feel about themselves and their lives?

Because Black women aren't a monolith, the answers to these questions vary greatly.

According to Nancy Boyd-Franklin, author of Black Families in Therapy, individuals exhibit a sense of greater power when they feel good about themselves and sustain a belief that religion and spirituality provide them with spiritual power. Empirical studies indicate that religion contributes positively to the mental well-being of individuals. Jacqueline Mattis and her colleagues note that what is not always clear is exactly how this positive change happens. Thorough interviews conducted with African American women can shed light on specific interventions or experiences in religion which contribute to positive mental well-being. In this study, I attempted to identify how religion contributed to positive mental well-being. A better understanding of this question can transform the implementation of policies regarding faith-based programs in local, state, and federal government. An exploration of the religiousness of African American women and its relationship to their mental well-being can shed light on what is needed for the all-around well-being for African American women.

I interviewed twenty women who received a flyer through various means such as social service organizations, nonprofit organizations, faith communities, and mental health centers. I also received interested persons from word-of-mouth referral. The flyer advertised that volunteers were needed for a research study on religion, mental well-being, and African American women. The semi-structured interviews included the following questions:

∗ Tell me about yourself.

∗ What do you know about mental well-being?

∗ Tell me about your mental well-being.

∗ How does religion connect with your mental well-being?

∗ Describe yourself when you are in a state of mental well-being.

∗ Share with me a story or a situation that helped you to understand better what mental well-being was for you as a woman.

∗ What is mental well-being to you, and how does it relate to you?

∗ Give me an example of how religion has affected you.

∗ Tell me about church in your life.

∗ Tell me about any negative experiences with religion.

∗ What have you learned about meditation?

∗ How does religion make you feel about yourself and your life?

∗ When was there a time you didn't feel good about you?

∗ What else would you share that is important for me to know?

∗ How does having faith in God help you in your life?

∗ What has not been helpful about religion?

The Black women's stories that I will present in this book are of every day ordinary women. They are women who show resilience despite finding themselves in stressful situations and sometimes traumatic circumstances. These women often find themselves pushing forward despite their arduous paths, often calling on their God. Despite their difficulties, they find themselves taking care of family and others in the community. They "make a way out of no way," and unbeknownst to them they are living womanist principles. As they survive and thrive, they are very clear about how they experience their mental well-being. They know the role that religion plays in their lives and whether it aids them or not, and they are also aware of how religion impacts how they feel about themselves.

Two

Liberation

My family experienced a difficult time when my young nephew died of a drug overdose. At the funeral, I was scheduled to read some remarks from the family. There were several men on the pulpit who were also giving remarks from the perspectives of how they knew my nephew. I was sitting on the front row with my family and when it was my turn, and I proceeded to take the steps up to the pulpit. There was a male usher on the side of me who kept calling me, saying, "Miss, Miss, Miss!" There was a podium on the floor, and it became apparent to me that this gentleman was trying to get my attention so that I could speak from the floor of the sanctuary. Evidently, this church did not allow women in the pulpit area. I continued up the steps and made my way to the large podium on the pulpit to give my remarks. As I stepped up, the pastor tentatively met me and handed me the microphone. I saw my brother smiling as he watched me from the pew because he knew that I was the first woman to step on this pulpit and speak and perhaps I was being a bit cheeky. In some way, I was aware that this was an act of defiance towards the sexism that is still prevalent in some Black churches today. Later, several older women smiled and patted me on the back as they told me how they appreciated my words. In some way, this act of bold disobedience to the tradition of the church was a victory for them; they felt a sense of liberation for a few brief moments from the many ways they experience sexism in the church.

After four hundred years of chattel slavery and the subjugation of women since the beginning of time, Black women are finding a voice that announces their survival in a world that has hated them because they are Black and ignored them because they are women. Womanist theology and empowerment theory are the frameworks I used to study the experiences of Black women with religion and their mental well-being. Womanism as a discipline is known in the academy and the seminary, but in the community, Black women have often lived out "outrageous, audacious, courageous, and responsible behavior"—tenets of Womanism—in response to oppression in their lives, whether they knew what to call it or not.

I see myself as a privileged Black woman in that I have had the benefit of education and experiences. Working in the mental health arena, I have been very aware of racism in the treatment of Black patients and Black women. As a religious professional, I have been very aware of sexism in the Black Church. Many barriers have been broken regarding sexism in the church, but in too many instances, circumstances remain the same. Womanism promotes the notion and belief that Black women are equally valid, and that their level of self-respect has much to do with their own sense of self-love.

As a Black woman who has traversed both the professional mental health community and the Black Church, the notion of Womanism speaks to me right where I live. Womanist theology is a theology of liberation. It is done by Black women in the context of African American community life, religion, and spirituality. As a Black woman, I too struggle for survival, liberation, and wholeness in my day-to-day life. Womanist theology emerges out of day-to-day struggles of Black women, including experiences with the unjust exercise of authority or power over them, discrimination based on their social class, prejudice and racism, and gender-based discrimination. These intersecting systems of discrimination challenge me as a Black woman and where I see God and God's action in my life. Despite experiencing sexual abuse as a young child, despite experiencing racism in the classroom in all White schools in my teenage years, despite coming from a family that struggled financially, I can reflect and see God's action in my life. I experience God not only as a liberator, but also as a sustainer in that God opens doors where there are only walls for me. Many Black women can identify with this experience. Womanist theology focuses on unity and holistic well-being of the entire Black community and with this consciousness comes understanding and a new sense of ability for Black women. It gives me significance in my life and allows me to try to be all that God wants me to be knowing that God rescues me and helps me in my day-to-day life.

African American women religious scholars developed womanist theological thought. Previously, the assessment and insight of Black women were absent from both Black theology and feminist theological scholarship. Alice Walker described a womanist as a black feminist or feminist of color: "Womanist behavior was seen as outrageous, audacious, courageous, or willful behavior. Wanting to know more and in greater depth than is considered 'good' for one. Interested in grown-up doings. Acting grown up. Being grown up."

Womanist theology is a reply to sexism in Black theology and racism in feminist theology. Since the advent of womanist theology, womanist thought has found its way into every academic discipline where there is a need for liberation and empowerment for women of color. In the academy outside of theological studies, the same construct is called womanist theory.

Womanist theology is a part of the framework supporting this study. It examines the relationships between gender, class, race, racism, sexism, and power and is exceptionally pertinent to this study because it portrays how African American women's lives are shaped by the systemic oppression within American society that affects the empowerment of African American women. As the work of womanist theologian Monica Coleman demonstrates, it examines "the social construction of black womanhood in relation to the African American community and religious concepts."

Layli Phillips proposed five essential components of womanist theology: a) It is anti-oppression. It is identified with liberation ventures of all kinds and supports the liberation of all humankind from all types of oppression. b) It is vernacular. Womanism is identified with "the everyday"—everyday people and everyday life; grassroots diversity is celebrated. c) It is non-ideological. Womanism is not about building lines of demarcation, but about building structures of inclusiveness and positive interrelationships. d) It is communitarian. Womanism views "commonweal" as the goal of social change. Commonweal is the state of collective well-being, the optimization of well-being for all members of the community. e) It is spiritualized. Womanism explicitly accepts a spiritual/transcendental sphere in which all of life and the material world are intertwined. Taken together, the components of womanism lead to improved relationships.

According to Corliss Heath, womanism seeks to reconcile three relationships: 1) the relationship between people from different groups, 2) the relationship between people and the environment/nature, and 3) the relationship between people and the spiritual. A womanist framework examines how to strengthen relationships and assists in understanding the resilience and empowerment of African American women within an oppressed society, including the impact of religion on their lives. This more holistic and inclusive view can only bring health and wholeness to the African American community.

As noted, the term "womanist" was coined by the Pulitzer Prize winning novelist Alice Walker. Well known in religious scholarship is Walker's explanation that a womanist is "a woman who loves other women, sexually and/or non-sexually. It focuses on the whole of women's relationships and does not discriminate. Womanism appreciates and prefers women's culture and is committed to survival and wholeness of entire people, male and female."

In womanist thought, the knowledge of God develops from the struggle for liberation of Black women and their community. A Black woman's many roles work together to unite the community in affirming freedom and life, thereby bringing wholeness to the entire community. Whereas some feminist thought is concerned mostly with women as individuals, womanism goes beyond Black women's self-liberation to the liberation and well-being of the entire community.

Empowerment is closely aligned with womanism. In her book *Black Empowerment: Social Work in Oppressed Communities*, Barbara Bryant Solomon examines the powerlessness of individuals and groups, especially African Americans, where esteemed roles, identities, and resources are absent. She sees empowerment as a goal for persons in stigmatized groups, such as African American women, who are not valued due to marginalization, stigma, and the effects of pervasive discriminatory practices.

As a result of generations of discriminatory practices, individuals in general, and African Americans in particular, are left in paralyzing conditions, which, Solomon argued, is by design. One effect of powerlessness in Solomon's analysis is the inability to cope with feelings, abilities, information, and or material resources in a manner that allows a person to function in a way that garners them respect and personal fulfillment.

Solomon also contends that there are indirect power blocks that affect African Americans who are poor and live in the inner cities of the United States. The primary blocks come from negative values that are integrated into the family and prevent growth of personal resources and positive self-concepts. The primary blocks lead to a lack of interpersonal and technical skills that result in a decreased ability to perform in social roles.

Experience shows that in today's culture, African Americans who are poor and disenfranchised continue to experience power blocks. In cities all over America, gentrification as well as disproportionate incarceration of African Americans contribute to these power blocks in various ways as African Americans lose their homes, their jobs, and are pushed out of urban areas due to increases in the cost of living in the city. The example of Flint, Michigan is a poignant illustration of these power blocks: its residents, forty percent of whom are living below the official poverty line, have been physically affected by high levels of lead in their water which is showing up in their children's blood samples.

African Americans in the urban context are often recognized as a marginalized population with low or no income, poor education, and inadequate resources. Their impoverished environment contributes to this population's lack of empowerment in their communities. The inability of individuals to become empowered in their communities is illustrated by Nancy Boyd-Franklin's concept of the victim system. Boyd-Franklin's victim system refers to a twelve-stage process:

* A community with barriers to opportunities and education
* Limited chances of achievement, employment, and attainment of skills
* Poverty
* Stress in relationships
* Inadequate performance of family roles
* Problems in individual growth and development
* Families unable to meet their own needs
* Inability to organize or improve their communities
* Communities have limited resources (jobs, education, housing)
* Communities are unable to support families
* Communities become a disorganizing influence, a breeder of crime and pathology
* Powerlessness

Barbara Solomon perceived empowerment as a process of establishing effective support systems for those who have been blocked from attaining their personal or collective goals. Empowerment can work to liberate and support those who have been marginalized and discriminated against. Social workers and clinicians can contribute to empowerment when they undertake practices that identify an individual's power blocks and help diminish powerlessness.

Building on Solomon's work, Lorraine Gutierrez claimed, "empowerment is a process of increasing personal, interpersonal, or political power so that individuals can take action to improve their life situations." It requires challenging oppression, obtaining needed resources, defining needs, and developing one's own center of control. Gutierrez examined the experience of "double jeopardy" for persons who are both women and persons of color. Compared to White women, women of color earn less money and are under-represented in positions of power in government and the private market. She contended that powerlessness has a specific physical and emotional impact in the lives of women of color. According to the National Women's Law Center, African American women who worked full-time year-round were receiving only sixty cents per dollar of what was paid to their White, non-Hispanic counterparts. In addition, African American women had the largest wage gap of all groups. African American women's struggle with racism, sexism, poverty, and the mental health difficulties that these issues engender points to a need for empowerment of these women in their day-to-day lives.

Empowerment theory has a history in the field of community organizing. Organizing can also affect individual empowerment, just as individual empowerment can affect the group. It is interesting to note that community organizing is often facilitated through faith communities. Members of churches and other faith traditions use their faith to propel them to address issues such as poverty, unemployment, and unfair government practices. These problematic issues disproportionately disenfranchise African American women, and frequently the participants of the community actions are overwhelmingly African American women who are trying to improve their lives.

Cheryl Holcomb-McCoy proposed that the triple oppression that African American females experience—being female, African American, and often poor or working class—has a detrimental effect on African American girls. She asserts that the development of empowerment groups for these girls cannot be effective without acknowledging the commonality of race, gender, and class oppression, including the legacy of struggle for African American females. In addition, these groups must have an African American female counselor as part of the leadership team in order for girls to identify with her and move forward to empowerment. African American girls become African American women whose experiences then influence the community.

Womanist theology is often influenced by religion, especially the Black Church. It is concrete in that it is effected by Black women, and reflects the active commitment of their struggle for survival, liberation, and wholeness in their daily lives. The questions "who is God for me," and "how does God function in my life" are important questions for Black women. These are questions that may easily find themselves as the focus of any counseling or therapy session.

Equally as important is the question, "how might I have peace and be delivered from those things that oppress me in my life?"

The questions that Black women bring forward can cause them to contemplate how religion can move them to a deeper sense of spirituality. This spirituality can give them an inner strength, and their struggle becomes a process of liberating reflection and action. This means that when women start to think differently, they often feel differently and become empowered to take action that is helpful to them.

As we think of the empowerment of Black women, both religion and empowerment theory have some similarities. Empowerment theory advocates for effective support systems to help those who are oppressed and marginalized. In religion, the Black church has established various support systems. Worship services, Bible studies, women's ministries, and support groups function to inspire, strengthen, guide, and help women and others feel better about themselves which can help them to take action that will benefit them. Empowerment theory promotes increasing both personal and political power. When individuals within the church feel personally empowered by what the church shares with them, this can help the church to increase its own political power. I am aware of churches involved in community organizing to develop and get jobs for people, to provide affordable housing for the poor, to provide tangible resources like increasing the number of "violence interrupters" in the community, to send mental health providers for those in a crisis in response to 911 calls, to invest in evidence-based culturally competent behavioral health and wellness services, and to promote holistic public health approaches to school safety that is relational, racially just, restorative, trauma responsive, and trauma informed. This means church members within religious institutions often become involved politically to effect change. When these kinds of activities are happening, religious institutions run parallel with empowerment theory. Individual empowerment within religious institutions gives way to group empowerment and moves people to act to improve their life situation. The people identify the power blocks and diminish their powerlessness in the places where they have been marginalized and discriminated against.

Understanding that womanism is "spiritualized" is understanding that all aspects of life, the transcendent and the world, are intertwined with one another. Even if one is not religious, it would be beneficial for Black women to get curious about connecting their own spirit with "The Spirit" if they want to be empowered. It became clear to me that the more I reflected on God and how the Spirit "stirred me and disturbed me," and compelled me to change and grow, the more I was empowered to improve life for myself, and for my community.

Womanist theology and empowerment theory are similar frameworks in that both are anti-oppressionist. Womanist theology focuses on gender and race discrimination of Black women and empowerment theory focuses on all who are stigmatized and marginalized. The components of realized empowerment theory are personal power is increased, interpersonal power is increased, and political power is increased. When womanist theology materializes, there is inclusivity, wholeness, empowerment, social change, liberation, well-being, concern for all humanity, dialogue, positive interrelations, and diversity.

Standing in the pulpit at my nephew's funeral, I experienced the full force of womanism and empowerment. Nevertheless, serving as a Black woman pastor and a psychotherapist who has worked with many Black women over the years has given me an understanding of the struggles that ordinary Black women endure and their means of engaging the world in ways that can bring them benefit and relief. However, I have also been able to witness how women, despite their discrimination and oppression, have been able to become empowered to have a better life and bring change to the family and her community.

Three

Coping

I was scheduled to see Mary Beth at ten o'clock in the morning. She lived in a poor part of town in a brick apartment building where there were no trees and no grass, only dirt. As I approached the building, three women were on the step already drinking beer this time of the day. They were laughing and talking loudly and did not move as they saw me coming. I said, "Good morning," they responded, "Good morning" but still did not move. I had to step on the small stoop from the side. As I entered the building, there was trash on the floor and the foyer did not appear to have been swept for some time. Mary Beth lived on the first floor; her apartment was the first one to the left as I entered. I knocked on the door with the door knocker and a tall thin man looking to be in his forties opened the door. I said good morning and told him I had an appointment with Mary Beth. He said, "Come on in, she's expecting you." I followed the man into a small dark room. I felt a little wary until I saw Mary Beth sitting in a chair with an oxygen tube in her nose and a bright smile. I immediately relaxed when I experienced her welcoming smile. She had long hair and a pretty face and looked younger than her forty-four years. The apartment smelled flowery like they had just sprayed air freshener. She said, "You met my husband." She seemed to know that there were people sitting on the stoop and apologetically explained that there were always people out there making noise, drinking, and doing drugs. She said she couldn't wait till she could move.

Mary Beth contracted HIV/AIDS at the age of eighteen and has been living with it for twenty-five years. She is also a domestic abuse survivor. She admitted to suffering post-traumatic stress disorder (PTSD) because of her abuse and the stigma she suffered from having AIDS. It appears that for most of her life, she has been adjusting to mental and physical illness while living in poverty and raising two children. She is aware of her mental illness and her physical illness as well as the contributing factors of her history of domestic violence, and her impoverished environment, which has led to her experiencing anxiety and panic attacks; however, she feels that she has learned to manage well despite the complexities of her life. Although Mary Beth had faced several challenges, she recently married and finds comfort, care, and love in this relationship. It has been her religiosity that has allowed her to maintain stability in her life. She is able to meditate and pray in both her clinical appointments at her agency, as well as in her worship at church. Several of her church members are living with AIDS, including her pastor:

Mary Beth receives SSI for physical disability. She has two adult children and two grandchildren. She receives medical and behavioral health services in a clinic. She sees her progress in her physical health as interventions by God because of her deep belief. She said:

> I am forty-four years old, I have two grown children, twenty-three and twenty-four, and two grandchildren, one who came six weeks ago. I go to a group for HIV support, meditation groups and mental health support groups. The church, God, is a big part of my life because I was positive since I was eighteen, those twenty-five years. Spirituality is a big part of my life. I'm

> married for about two years but I have been with my soul mate for a total of nine years. I'm just blessed to be alive. Because when they told me I was positive at eighteen they said I had six months to live. I was pregnant at the time, but I had no idea that I was going to see my children grow up and I will see grandchildren. God has been really good to me in spite of.

Mary Beth continues to see God as a healer even when she is going through difficulty. She feels that God will heal her even though she is going through arduous times because of what she has interpreted as God's action in the past.

> Just recently I got on oxygen because I kept getting pneumonia and I have been oxygenated before about ten years ago and then I got off of it. I basically have gotten back on but it's only temporarily, God is a healer. He has healed me before from it so He will do it again, so I'm not worried about it. I have a lot of doctors looking after me so spiritually, mentally, emotionally, physically I have to take care of all aspects of my life in order to stay whole and complete. God gives me hope, it makes me know there is a power bigger than me that's taking care of me despite of whatever the doctors are saying. I've seen many people pass away from the virus and God has spared me and given me as I said grandbabies now. I have taken medications as I'm supposed to, I pray, I meditate, I go to church just knowing that He is there with me.

Mary Beth indicates that because of what God has done in the past for her, she has hope. She sees her life as God's intervention, saving her despite what doctors have said. She is faithful in using her religious resources and her medicine, cooperating with God's action in her life.

> I had pneumonia and had acute sinusitis and the antibiotics didn't work. The first three days I got a fever, I was kind of delirious. I changed the antibiotics to Cipro. Cipro worked that's when they put me on oxygen. They had me walking and they said my oxygen levels went down to like eighty so they put me on oxygen. I was a little disturbed at first but then I remembered, wait a minute, hold up, I've been here ten years ago, and I was on oxygen and God got me off oxygen. There is

> no need to fret, no need to worry, this is all temporary. Maybe
> He needs you to slow down a little bit to take care of yourself,
> so I take it as He is saying, I've got you.

Mary Beth is interpreting what is happening to her through her spirituality. She does some reflection and feels that what is happening to her is for her good because God needs her to slow down, and she feels good about this.

> But in doing that, being in a hospital made me realize that I have
> really bad allergies, so I think I'm going to have to get a shot
> every week. Then my sinus infections cause the pneumonias
> so what we are going to do with the sinus infection is they are
> going to go in and do some reconstruction in my sinuses to
> open my sinuses up so that I wouldn't get pneumonia. It was
> all a blessing to tell you the truth, to figure out all these things
> would happen with me, and they are fixable. God just took the
> situation that I thought was bad in the hospital and reveals some
> things that's going to heal me, it was God's way of healing me.

Again, Mary Beth interprets what she thought was injurious as a blessing and feels this is God's action in moving to heal her. She is using her interpretation of God's action in her life as a mechanism that helps her cope with her physical ailments. She is using her religious beliefs to maintain a sense of well-being. Religion has been used by many to survive and understand difficulty in their lives. It helps them to interpret and manage their daily difficulties and can bring them a sense of meaning. When faced with seemingly impossible situations, God creates an understanding, solution, or path where none existed before. Both research and theory suggest that religious coping is more likely to transpire in circumstances perceived as unmanageable. People have both natural and spiritual belief systems within them that tend to work together to help them understand and deal with life's challenges. How one is able to use religious coping varies by individual traits and social location. Religious coping helps in satisfying the human need for meaning and purpose of life.

Mary Beth really wants to move out of the neighborhood she is in. She is looking for a three-bedroom house in another part of the city where there is no violence, and it is peaceful. She has not been able to find this with her Section 8 voucher. It has been her faith and her spirituality that allows her to cope with her trauma and to continue living where she is. She uses her "tools" that she has learned both in the clinic where they have taught her meditation, and her church does meditation with deep breathing and soft music at the start of their service. Meditation, prayer, and attending church allow her to deepen her faith and develop a sense of peace amid the turmoil of the people who live around her and her environment.

Many African Americans rely on religion to cope with life's challenges and for various other reasons. Using religious resources as tools such as prayer, attending church, support from church members, reading religious material, meditation, yoga, attending religious activities among other resources can help to give a sense of confidence and peace as individuals negotiate their lives.

Individual experience and social location determine how individuals perceive their life. For example, African American caregivers will often report feeling inner strength and acceptance from God as they help those who need physical assistance and care. Their religious involvement helps them to perceive their work as service to God, whereas Whites may perceive their caregiving as stressful and overwhelming. African Americans will often use their religious coping skills when they are in ill health and may call on their pastors to pray for them. These clergy often find themselves attending to a myriad of concerns in their congregations and community. Whether it is unemployment, legal problems, marital and family problems, depression, substance abuse, alcoholism, teenage pregnancy, or other concerns, pastors often find themselves addressing the same problems that mental health professionals address. Depending on their education, some may refer to mental health professionals, and others may see mental health problems as religious problems and encourage prayer and worship attendance.

Religion often becomes more pertinent when individuals are experiencing problems in their lives. Faith has been a significant source of strength for African Americans when facing a crisis. Kenneth Pargament and his colleagues found that the use of religious resources has been effective in the face of psychological and emotional illness. In particular, he determined that certain coping mechanisms can be helpful, such as seeking spiritual support, re-evaluating one's religious beliefs or practices, considering new experiences or challenges, forgiving others on the basis of one's religious beliefs or practices, providing within a religious framework, and seeking clergy support.

Participation in religion has also been helpful in preventing anxiety and distress. Janice Bowie and her colleagues did a study looking at coping styles and breast cancer. They identified several coping styles:

* Self-Directing: God gives individuals the abilities to take care of their own problems.

* Deferring: Surrender to God, God will fix it as persons wait patiently.

* Collaborative: God is a partner and together God and the individual will work it out.

The researchers found that individuals who totally accepted their church's teaching and attended churches that were more charismatic and believed in divine healing had lower levels of anxiety. Therefore, a coping style that is deferring rather than self-directing or collaborative suggests how religion is helpful in the lives of Black women. There can be some overlap between the collaborative and deferring style, but not with the self-directed style.

Using these coping styles, another study in a Black Baptist congregation examined whether a belief in one's personal internal control—meaning the individual's ability to regulate their own behavior, actions and outcomes—or God's control most contributed to a religious person's sense of purpose in life. They found that having a strong belief in God's being in control did not prevent one's own personal internal control. Laurence Jackson and Robert Coursey determined that while the deferring style of coping was important for African Americans, it overlapped with the collaborative style. The authors felt that useful coping is effected by personal control through God instead of believing in an all controlling God.

Mary Beth believed that despite what the doctors were saying regarding her illness, God would heal her and bring her through. At the same time, however, she cooperated with treatment, went to the clinic, and got physical and mental health care. She went to her church, which bolstered her spirituality. She cooperated with her own healing. She believed that God is a healer, and deferred to God in that respect, but at the same time, she collaborated by seeing her physical and mental health providers and practicing her religion. In short, her effective coping was achieved by her own personal control through God. She did not believe that God would spontaneously heal her; rather, she cooperated with the resources offered and felt more in control of herself and had better well-being.

Despite this, being religious has not always helped individuals. Sometimes, religious resources such as sermons, reading religious material, or church, can have a negative slant and may make individuals feel punished or abandoned by God. This is based on their belief that they will be punished for their sin, or that God has left them. Feeling that God is absent can happen when one is deeply grieving. When grieving the death of someone, a condition can develop called complicated grief, in which intense and prolonged emotional pain makes it difficult for individuals to recover from the loss and get back to living their own lives. In studying forty-eight African American homicide survivors, Laurie Burke and her colleagues found that those with complicated grief had negative religious coping, which means that they may have harbored thoughts of anger towards God or their faith community. They may have felt abandoned by God and felt no sense of spirituality. They often could not go on with their normal activities of daily living. Many of the African American homicide survivors exhibited an intensifying spiritual crisis over a period of six or more months instead of a gradual recovery.

Complicated grief could progress into complicated spiritual grief, in which grief instigates a spiritual crisis so intense that the individual cannot reestablish a spiritual life after the loss. This is often accompanied by a sense of contention, conflict, distance from God, and, at times, distance from members of one's spiritual community. A significant number of African American homicide survivors in this study could find no meaning in their situation and therefore could develop no coping skills. Burke acknowledged Kenneth Pargament and his colleagues' five key religious functions for individuals.

* Spiritual coping to find meaning
* Gain control of a stressful situation
* Gain God's comfort and closeness

* Gain intimacy with others
* Achieve a life transformation

It is clear, however, that some individuals benefit from spiritual struggles, through which they gain inner strength and coping skills. On the other hand, there are some who never develop positive coping skills because of the depth of their pain, trauma, and crisis, and the inability to find meaning in it. This is where clinicians can assist faith communities to be more aware of the members when they are going through extreme struggle so that helpful care may be given. African Americans tend to have strong religious connections; however, stereotypes need to be avoided so that people can be met at their own point of need.

Mental and physical illness can have devastating effects on individuals, the family, and the community. The lives of African American women are sometimes complicated by mental illness and physical instability. However, frequently, these women assess their lives positively despite mental health and physical health challenges. Mary Beth describes many of the traumas and difficulties of her life. As she shares what domestic violence has done to her, she also explains that her environment and poor housing re-traumatize her and add to her stress. Safe and proper housing is important for positive mental well-being.

> I have anxiety. I was in a domestic violence relationship for eight years, so I have had very high anxiety to a point of panic attacks. I have depression, but I haven't been depressed in over a year. I take medication. I have insomnia, so I take medication for sleep. Right now my mental well-being is very stable. I do have some phobias because of the domestic violence . . . Because of the environment that I live in, and, you see, they are out there all the time drinking, drugging, cursing, fussing, cutting each other, the ambulance is coming, and it brings back the domestic violence that I have been through . . . I have flashbacks when I hear them cutting each other, and I have called the police to stop them.

Mary Beth goes on to say that she has to use specific resources and interventions to aid in her mental well-being. She talks about engaging in meditation with her psychiatrist and in the context of worship at church. Much of her life revolves around keeping herself physically and mentally well.

> God has kept me still and peaceful as much as possible, but I also have to use my tools, meditate, pray, deep breathing that also has decreased the size of my anxiety, post-traumatic stress disorder, and working with my therapist, taking my medication.

Amongst the other women I spoke with, Mary Beth was not the only one with a perception of viewing religion through a mental health lens. When I first met Becky, I knocked on her door and her adult son opened the door and said, "She's here!" He let me in, and Becky said, "Oh Good, you have the gift card right?" She was referring to the fact that each person interviewed would get a $25 gift card. I was taken aback and said that I would give it to her at the end of the interview. She said, "Oh never mind that, just give it to my son." Becky's adult son and daughter were standing looking at me, so I reluctantly gave it to him. After this, Becky had several instructions for them to go to someone's house, pick them up, go to the store, and get several items. She was talking very fast, and I felt that my head was spinning. I was still standing in her neat but small apartment when she said, "Okay come on make yourself at home, sit down what you want to ask me?" She had a big grin on her face and I finally breathed and relaxed so I could start the interview. She was very happy to talk and share her story.

Becky stated that she was bipolar and attended a mental health clinic. She said she was forty-three years old and she had five children and two beautiful grandkids. She has been attending her church for thirteen years and has been a minister in her church for eight years. She claims that she ministers to many people in her life. Becky receives disability insurance payments; she is tall and obese and walks with a cane. Becky shared that she had been physically, sexually, and emotionally abused as a child and had also been addicted to drugs. Becky felt that it was the mental health center and God who rescued her in her life and continues to keep her.

"Like I said, He [God] kept me. You will see, you know a lot of people, if you go to the. . . or . . . or . . . , these are the real mental health agencies . . . One thing for certain and two things for sure, you always hear them talking about God."

In describing her mental well-being, Becky also mentions the state of her mental health and how she attends an agency to effect mental well-being. She directly connects mental well-being with getting help for mental health issues. She basically defines mental well-being as going to an agency and seeing mental health clinicians. She also sees participating in spiritual disciplines as a part of keeping herself mentally well. She appears proud of the fact that she can describe herself as having mental well-being because she goes to a behavioral health agency and is very connected to God.

> I do have mental health issues I go to . . . for my mental health. I'm diagnosed with mainly depression. That means I have my highs and lows. When I feel myself going into one of my episodes I know how to reach out for help. I pray on a daily basis; I know without God I'm nothing. Without Him, I can do nothing. I'm very spiritually connected to him. I would say mental well-being is where, though you do have mental issues or a mental illness and you are connected with an agency that can help you control that if it's medication wise, therapy wise, whatever it is, you know, you are working on it, you're tapped into it. Yes, I do, yes, I feel as though I do, I have mental well-being.

Despite instances of extreme trauma in their lives, Becky and Mary Beth felt it was their connection and involvement in religion that helped them to negotiate their day-to-day lives. By meticulously sharing their life stories, they allow us to understand not only how they experienced mental illness and mental health diagnoses, but how their understanding of religion allowed them to cope daily with their challenges and empower them in their lives.

Becky has had to cope with early trauma in her life. She described raising herself while going through several rapes in her life starting at eight years old. Her mother was mentally ill as was her grandmother, but Becky stated they never got help. Her family also had a history of drug abuse and alcoholism. Becky described not really having a childhood because she had to care for her siblings due to the fact that her mother and the mother's cadre of boyfriends were using drugs and alcohol. For Becky to have a relationship with her mother, she began doing drugs with her. During this time, she tried to end her life by suicide twice. It was then that she entered a drug treatment program and her life changed. She describes her five children as also having drug-related issues and mental health issues.

> Yes, there was a time in my life where I have a lot of child abuse issues and stuff and sexual abuse as a child. I turned to the street drugs to medicate myself, so I wouldn't feel at one time in my life. During that time no I was not under nobody's care, I wasn't getting no mental health none of that.

Becky feels that it has been God who has kept her because throughout her life, while difficulties were present, she still went to church, and she feels it is God who has kept her and taken care of her.

> I just know I'm so grateful. God has really sustained me, and these are really tears of gratefulness. Because I can look back and see where He brought me from all the hurdles that He has walked me over when I didn't think it was no way that I was going to make it through He was there. When I didn't have nobody, He was there. He never left me; He never forsake me. I just thank God because if it wasn't for God where would I be?

Like Becky, Mary Beth shared how important God was to her and how God helped her in her process of recovering from mental health problems and medical illnesses. She asserts that she needed to address her physical, emotional, and spiritual issues. She feels she gets these issues addressed in the clinic she attends where she sees a medical doctor, a psychiatrist and a therapist. She also attributes her wholeness to attending church where meditation is practiced, and her pastor can identify with her because he has AIDS.

As individuals we are body, mind, and spirit. To be whole, all the parts of us need to be addressed and fed. Both women share a long history of religion and spirituality but came to a knowledge that their mental health issues needed to be addressed by professionals in the mental health community. They acknowledge that it is the combination of these modalities that has brought forth their wholeness. It is my opinion that when there is undue stress and trauma, having faith and trust in God is good, but one also needs their state of mind and mental health issues to be addressed to be whole. It was only when these women were able to add mental health care to their religion and spirituality that they felt relief, peace, and mental well-being.

Some years ago, a mother brought her young adult daughter to me and the mother and the daughter, who were very devout Christians, asked if I could do an exorcism. The daughter was experiencing auditory hallucinations—voices that were calling her names and telling her terrible things about herself. In assessment, her appearance was disheveled, she was agitated, but her mood was depressed. She had delusions saying that if I coughed, she knew that was the devil. The mother and daughter said they wanted an exorcism because they knew a demon was in this young girl. I scheduled another appointment with the daughter who came by herself this time. I explained to her that I did not do exorcisms. I believed that God used people to treat and heal, and explained that she may have schizophrenia that was treatable with medication. I met with her several times, and it appeared she had gained some trust in me. I took her to a psychiatrist that I referred clients to, and he started her on medication. Within two months she no longer heard voices, her mood was much better, the delusions were gone, and she not only was coming to worship, but she joined the choir. She talked about how God used me to take her to the psychiatrist to get medicine that made her feel and function better.

This young woman's religion initially brought her to me, a psychotherapist and a pastor. She saw me as a religion-based pastor who could spiritually heal her. But it was in providing mental health services, both counseling and medication management through a psychiatrist, that brought her relief. In other words, both religion and mental health services that brought her mental well-being.

Coping mechanisms are very helpful for me to eliminate my stress. I became an advocate for taking care of self, not just for my clients, but for myself. It's crucial for Black women to prioritize self-care since they often must deal with numerous stressors. The use of coping tools is helpful for these stressors. When you feel yourself experiencing anxiety, or feel very low or depressed, or even other symptoms that appear to impact your behavior and internal sense of peace, even though you may pray and practice spiritual disciplines, these stories help to illustrate that seeking mental health care from a clinician may be what is needed to become whole.

Four

Hope in the Face of Hardship

When I think of hope, I think of the Reverend Jessie Jackson's mantra to "keep hope alive!" He wanted people to believe that change could come, that inclusivity of all voices in the nation was a possibility, and that common ground for all people in the United States was conceivable. I also think of the scripture from Hebrews 11:1: "Now faith is the substance of things hoped for, the evidence of things not seen"—things that are "not yet." The verse urges us to deeply believe in God and God's promises, and to demonstrate faith even though we might not see the realization of those promise. The New Oxford American Dictionary defines hope as "a feeling of expectation and desire for a certain thing to happen."

For me, hope is one of the positive virtues of the Christian faith that I hang my hat on. I hoped one day I would marry; I hoped

45

when I was in seminary, I would get ordained; I hoped my children would go to college. When I hoped, it had not yet happened. I knew these things were a possibility, and indeed did happen, but at the time I hoped, they were "not yet." I hoped I would be "called" to a particular church as pastor; it did not happen when I wanted it to, but I still had hope until it actually happened.

In the African American community, hope is something that is born of centuries of despair and dehumanization as well as the tragic sense of life. Rev. Dr. Martin Luther King, Jr. promoted hope in the Black community, but it was often disappointing and not realized. It was a discipline that King saw people needed to keep executing. This hope was related to suffering, and even though one may not achieve all the relief from suffering in life, this hope can enable people to go forward and do meaningful work.

Hope for Black women allows women to "keep on keeping on." Mary Beth was hoping for a new home in another part of her city where these opportunities were few and far between, but she continued to hope. Becky hoped she would continue to have mental well-being so she continued going to her clinic. Black women hope their children are not gunned down by police even as this is happening in our country seemingly every day. It is the hopes and dreams of African American people that have allowed this population to make gains of getting good jobs, education, and good homes. At the same time, things remain the same: for instance, African American women earn sixty cents on the dollar compared with their white male counterparts. Black mothers have hopes for their children, but often in poor Black communities there are barriers to opportunity, education, and resources that limit chances for realization of goals, employment, and the ability to attain skills.

Yet despite all of this, Black women do not totally lose their hope in the midst of difficulty. In a study of ten-week interventions with suicidal African American women who had experienced intimate partner abuse, Natalie Arnette found that when women had low levels of hopelessness, they experienced significantly higher levels of existential well-being after a ten-week intervention. Furthermore, those with positive religious coping had higher levels of religious well-being after a ten-week intervention. In short, lower levels of hopelessness and positive religious coping predicted spiritual well-being. Researchers pointed out that for women who are involved in faith communities, the response to domestic violence from the Black Church has been less than adequate with respect to needed education and alternative biblical interpretation to assist survivors in seeking help and empowerment.

Religion and spirituality's role is to engender hope, confidence, and expectation in daily life. Research shows that African Americans are more likely to receive screenings and develop positive health behaviors when receiving messages of hope. However, negative messaging to African American women fosters a sense of hopelessness instead of optimism, and African American and Hispanic women are exposed disproportionately to advertisements that perpetuate negative health effects, diminished spiritual well-being, decreased hope, and increased depression. Negative media messages can involve harmful stereotypes, such as portraying them as overly aggressive, hypersexualized, or unintelligent. This type of messaging can have detrimental effects on women's mental health, self-esteem, and overall well-being. It can also contribute to the marginalization and discrimination that Black women face in our society. This lack of constructiveness with an unhealthy, unbalanced, negative portrait of Black women contributes to health disparities in Black women leading to despair and lack of hope. It is important to challenge and counteract these negative portrayals by promoting diverse and empowering representations of African American women in the media. It is the positive portrayals that can bring hope to Black women.

Although the Black Church brings messages of hope, it can also contribute to shame and stigma. One area in which the church has contributed to both shame and stigma, thus negatively affecting spiritual well-being, is in its attitude about sexually transmitted diseases and sexuality in general. The church often does not address sex at all except to say "don't do it" if you are single and female, while subjecting girls to stereotypes and stigma. In contrast, men's behavior is often approached with an attitude of "boys will be boys," thus sparing them the stigma. Only in recent years have some aspects of the Black Church begun to advocate for sex education, use of condoms, and safe sex. It wasn't long ago that young women were ostracized and persecuted for becoming pregnant out of wedlock.

Participation in an ethic of resistance by promoting positive health messages of support, hope, and transformation can empower African American women. This means that there are values that guide individuals or communities in their resistance against oppression and injustice. It involves actively challenging and opposing systems of power and advocating for social change. An ethic of resistance offers transformative language, liberating education, and intergenerational stories of health and resiliency and helps African American women to make better choices and change their behavior, thus increasing positive spiritual well-being. Examining media messages and their impact on the mental health of African American women is necessary to provide a holistic model for healthy and effective health interventions.

Positive messages of hope go hand in hand with a sense of justice and feeling of well-being in positive mental health. Ann Fisher and Kenna Bolton Holz have demonstrated that women's personal experiences with sexism are connected to their beliefs about justice. They hypothesized that the more injustice a woman perceived, the less fair her life appeared, and that a diminished sense of control would adversely affect her mental health, spiritual health, and well-being and strip her sense of hope. The authors concluded that discrimination of marginalized groups is a predictor of psychological distress. This discrimination also negatively affects women's spiritual health. Many participants referred to sexist events in their lives. The results were consistent with the claims of feminist scholars who contended that sexist prejudice and discrimination can influence the mental and spiritual health of women.

Interventions that will assist in eradicating prejudice and discrimination for women, especially marginalized women, are needed for empowerment. Womanist approaches for women of color that provide support, encouragement, and connection are necessary for empowerment. Carman Williams and Marsha Wiggins promoted a framework of womanist spirituality in counseling to counteract sexism and racism. Africentric and feminist approaches have been inadequate in addressing the complexities of Black women's oppression within the context of counseling. Womanist spirituality is needed to address the intricacies of sexism and racism. The authors pointed to sexism within Africentrism, and racism within the feminist movement. Neither of these directly addresses spirituality. Womanism encompasses spirituality as one of its components, and religion and spirituality is a core value of Black women.

It is important for counselors to recognize and embrace the various aspects of a person's identity such as spirituality, communalism, and emotional relatedness in order to help mitigate the psychological effects of racism and sexism. However, it is important to know that these approaches may not fully address the intersections of these oppressions or the multiple social stigmas. Womanist traditions can be used as a means of addressing multiple cultural stigmas (racism, sexism, classism, heterosexism). These traditions are powerful tools for clinical work with African American women. Spirituality is introduced and used holistically. Williams and Wiggins used a case study to illustrate that counselors who work with African American women must be culturally competent and recognize the bearing that racism, sexism, and other forms of marginalization have on this population.

Multiple stigmas have impacted African American women from their entry into the United States of America. Johnnie Hamilton-Mason emphasized the strengths of the African American woman who has been essential to the family and the community. Racism, sexism, gender inequality, and classism have affected African American women in various ways that haven't been given enough attention. There isn't enough reliable data on mental health among African American women because people haven't focused enough on gender and socio-economic differences. These differences place African American women at greater risk for stress factors related to physical and mental health.

A cousin of mine had several stress factors in her life. For many years she has been the caretaker of her mother, who has dementia and is 100 years old. She focused on the care of her mother and conscientiously tended to her mother's needs. When she started having some pain in her side, my cousin went to an urgent care center, which referred her to a nephrologist. The nephrologist determined that she had cancer in one of her kidneys and told her she needed to have her kidney removed. After she had her kidney removed, she was told she had to have one year of chemotherapy. When leaving the doctor's office my cousin was stressed and distraught, and she was run over by a car, which broke her ankle and wrist, forcing her to have surgery. As she was in the hospital that day she said, "I am ready to go home, I am ready to die." There were many factors multiplying her stress which brought her to a place of despair. As a Black woman and only child of her mother, she had the primary caretaking responsibility of her aged mother. This responsibility and all that had happened to her in a short period of time brought her to a place of despair. It was later as her children came to see her, and people called her to tell her they were praying for her, that her demeanor changed and her despair dissipated. It was the prayers within the context of religion that gave her hope.

I am amazed as I think about the multiple roles I have fulfilled in my life. I was a mother of three children, a wife, a pastor, a therapist with a practice, and an adjunct teacher at a university. As a Black woman, I felt I had to do everything well. Seeing clients, preparing for class, teaching class, cooking, going to children's events, preaching, doing Bible studies, visiting the sick—it was overwhelming. I was totally stressed out. As a clinician I knew what I would say to my clients, but for myself I could not see the forest for the trees. Finally, I knew I had to make some changes. The stress was making me very anxious and depressed. At that time, I closed my counseling practice until my children were grown and out of the house. I also stopped having responsibility for Bible study and I added some coping mechanisms. I engaged in mindfulness meditation practice and joined a yoga class with other Black women. I was more intentional about my devotional life, prayer, and journaling.

Johnnie Hamilton-Mason uses the precursor to womanist thought, Black feminist thought, to counter the image of the troubled and debased African American woman. She celebrates resiliency, spirituality, and connection with other women, the family, and community. The legacy of struggle and strength does not deny the diversity among Black women in class, ethnicity, education, socio-economic status, coping ability, and skills, among other factors. These stresses along with the intersections of oppression affect the mental health of Black women.

The circumstances faced by Black women are quite different to that of white women and Black men. Addressing the negative psychological stressors associated with the inequities that Black women experience necessitates positive interventions and supports.

A study of 259 white and Black women between the ages of thirty and sixty determined that physical activity, social support, and family structure increased psychological well-being. Physical activity helped to decrease depression, anxiety, and physical pain symptoms. Low physical activity and poor social and family support were factors that contributed to depressed mood. As the number of children in the home increased, Black women's mood also became more negative. To increase overall mood, Black women should take care to increase their physical activity, nurture their relationships with friends and family, and pay attention to their sense of well-being. Churches who partner with health organizations and provide health and exercise ministries using spiritual principles can improve the physical and psychological health of Black women.

Improving the psychological health of older African American women transitioning out of homelessness was the focus of a study by Olivia Washington and her colleagues. They identified five areas in determining how women had used faith and spirituality as coping mechanisms: (1) identity and beliefs; (2) affiliation and membership; (3) involvement; (4) practices; and (5) benefits. The authors concluded that faith and spirituality helped these African American women find support and hope. They defined faith as "the secure belief in God and a trusting acceptance of God's will," and spirituality as "a form of transpersonal expression of a person's hopes and aspirations." The functions of faith and spirituality, particularly prayer, were recognized as fundamental components of positive mental health efficacy. When older African American women used faith and spirituality as resources to safeguard against the adversities of homelessness, they developed internal strength, high levels of motivation, coping skills and compassion.

In summary, African American women have been discriminated against for their gender, race, and class. In addition to this historical trauma, their current challenges can continue to add to poor mental health. Multiple studies demonstrate that religious involvement and spirituality positively affect mental well-being. Even in the challenges of everyday life, African American women often see God amid their challenges and feel encouraged. As Black preachers will often say in their prayers, "If we never had problems, we wouldn't know that God could solve them." The coming together of religion and religious resources continues to engender hope, confidence, and expectations of justice in one's life even during times of despair.

Religion points to something greater than ourselves. It can move us into spirituality which promotes faith and helps individuals to deepen their relationship with God. Religion is often sought by Black women in search of hope from despair. Black women have been encouraged, strengthened, and enabled to push forward to both endure and alleviate their plight because they have used the resources of religion, which gives them a sense of optimism and confidence regarding positive possibilities.

The use of religious resources such as prayer, reading scripture and devotionals, going to worship, and meditation cultivates hope, which can propel women to action and empowerment when they have felt dejected and hopeless. This use of religious resources can move women, for example, to find a way out of domestic violence situations, or they can join a community organizing group and do something about injustices in their apartment complexes. When there is oppression in its many forms Black women have become empowered not only through prayer, but also meditation to give them a sense of peace during turmoil, reading sacred texts to inspire and embolden them, and participating in corporate worship which so often provides them pastoral care within a worshipping congregation. This practice of religion has allowed many women to experience success in bringing their hopes to fruition. When this happens, one hears them saying "Thank you Jesus!" or "Thanks be to God! God is blessing me!"

Another instance where the practice of religion has brought me hope and help is my participation with the Max Robinson Clinic. At the height of the AIDS crisis in the late nineties, I reached out to a clinic located in a poor Black neighborhood serving those who were struggling with HIV/AIDS. I wanted to offer whatever services might be helpful. I was aware of many Black churches that condemned those living with AIDS because they felt these individuals were either homosexual or were intravenous drug users. Many pastors and congregants in the church felt these individuals had sinned against God and were going to hell. The fact that many women contracted HIV from their sexual partners was not even an issue that the church addressed. There was a day treatment center in the clinic that held a community meeting twice a week. I attended the meetings for about three weeks wondering whether this group of Black men and women would be open to a spirituality group. I also wanted the group to get used to my presence. As I spent time with them and listened to them, I realized that they wanted a Bible study. I met with this community in our spirituality group for several years. New people would come into the group, and some would leave the group, especially if they found employment. As a group, the women and men talked about how they could not go back to their churches because of how the church felt about those living with AIDS and they could not go to their families because of how they treated them. The women shared that they could not share that they had AIDS because of the stigma. Before the clients were treated with HIV medication, they would sometimes develop infections that would show up on their face. This prevented them from going many places at all except the clinic. We spent time talking about the pain and shame of rejection by their families, friends, and churches. I remember being brought to tears and my heart aching for these women and men. So many of the women felt they had been blind-sided because they had no idea that their husbands or partners were either on the "down low" or were intravenous drug users.

My church had an AIDS ministry and tried to address the stigma. Several years earlier, this same clinic was located across the street from my church and on a very cold January the roof fell in, forcing the clinic to find a new place to practice. A community pastor referred them to our church, as we had a large building. They were supposed to be with us for two weeks, but they ended up being with us for two years. Some of the staff and clients started to attend worship. The hearts and minds of many of the church members were softened and changed, as we could no longer objectify those living with AIDS. We had developed relationships with them. The reality was, however, that the Black Church at large was closed off to this population. I remember praying for them every day. I wanted these individuals to know that God loved them and that they were children of God. I wanted them to know that their lives did have meaning. I kept their dilemma before my congregation. I had faith that God would intervene in the lives of these women and men. Within the Spirituality Group, once a month the clients would come to my church, and they would conduct a worship service themselves. Some served as the choir. There was someone who read scripture, someone presided, and someone gave the message. The others were the congregation who encouraged those who were serving. Staff also started coming to the spirituality group and to the monthly worship service. As we participated in our devotional Bible study, several persons disclosed how having AIDS was actually a blessing to them. They had been living in a manner with all kinds of risky behavior before AIDS entered their lives. As we studied the Bible and shared about their lives some started to reveal that they felt not only a call to healthy living and being careful about how they lived, but they developed an awareness of purpose in their lives. Before attending the Spirituality Group on a consistent basis, they had given up, and did not feel good about themselves. Now they had hope.

On one occasion in 2001, a reporter from the Blade, an LGBTQ weekly newspaper, wanted to write a story on the clinic. When she heard about the spirituality group, she asked if she could sit in and perhaps hear from the participants. They were eager to have her come. She wrote an article entitled "Covenant Baptist is 'ministry of liberation'" based on her visit. One of the members of the group was quoted in the article saying, "Rev. Chris always brings something to us with her presence and through scripture that makes you know everything is going to be all right." Stigma still prevailed, but I felt that God had answered my prayers because these individuals were able to feel better about themselves in their daily lives. As we prayed and discussed what the scriptures meant to us along with the devotional passage, people talked about what was going on in their lives, what the scripture was saying to them, and what they believed God for. It opened up the room to become a place where people could struggle with their lives. Everyone knew that what we talked about in our time together was confidential. It was a space where people could cry and be consoled and a space where we could pray for one another. It very much felt like a sacred space each time we met. I felt that God had answered my prayers. It felt like a place of justice.

The use of religious resources is helpful for people; however, I think that one also must be careful about how to view religion and its resources. There are some who believe that if they do everything that religion "requires" of them, their hopes and dreams should come true. When individuals are living their lives the way they think God wants them to—when they pray, participate in a ministry, and come to worship vowing never to miss a Sunday unless they are ill—they may become very disillusioned when some tragedy enters their lives or things don't turn out the way they want. It is almost as though they see God like Santa Claus. If they do all the religious activities and they are "good," then God will bless them and give them the desires of their hearts. When this doesn't happen persons can feel that they have been abandoned or rejected by God. They may say, "Why is God doing this to me! I have been good! I have been praying about this!" Their disappointment may lead to lose their faith and/or feel that God has disdain for them or has neglected them. They may feel like they don't know what they did wrong and don't know how to get in God's good grace again.

This is erroneous thinking. It is not about what you do in terms of practicing religion that puts you in right relationship with God. It is really about who you are. In the Christian faith, when inquiring what it is that one must do to please God, I am directed to John 6:28–29: "Then they asked him, 'What must we do to do the works God requires?' Jesus answered, 'The work is this: to believe in the one he has sent.'" Religion teaches one how to have an authentic relationship with God. This means that an inner transformation is necessary. To "believe" regardless of what is happening in one's life necessitates transcending circumstances and trusting that regardless of what is going on, God is with you and for you. Trusting and believing is paramount. As we look at the lives of Black women, the Black community at large, and their hardships, however, it becomes clear that belief by itself is not enough. For example, there is the issue of violence in the Black community in cities all over this nation; praying about it and worshipping by itself is not enough. Believing means you must also put your faith into action. Individual believers and churches can come together to do something about the violence in the community. They can bring the mayor of the city to large rallies where demands are made. These persons can attend community organizing training and advocate for interventions such as increasing the number of violence interrupters, dispatching mental health providers in response to 911 calls involving people in crisis, providing culturally competent health and wellness programs in the community, and adding racially just school safety programs. In other words, it is the belief that can then propel people to do something, to plan, and to develop steps to bring forth actual change and resolution because "faith by itself, if it does not have works is dead" (James 2:17 KJV).

Historically the Black Church has played a significant social, spiritual, and political role in the lives of African Americans and the Black community, but Black Americans today tend to say that predominantly Black churches have less influence now than they did fifty years ago. There are intellectual, social, and political challenges that impact both the Black Church and the church in general. The Covid-19 pandemic caused financial devastation for some Black churches. There has been a decline in church attendance, with a number of young people saying they are not religious, but they are spiritual. Some adhere to alternative forms of spirituality. Although African American congregants share that they hear topics that include politics, social justice, and race in the sermons preached in Black churches, these topics however, are a low priority for African Americans. They are more concerned about morality teaching, spiritual comfort, fellowship, assistance for the needy, housing and food, practical job and life skills, and racial pride.

There are areas the Black Church has not addressed on a large scale. With police violence and killing of Black men and women, more activism has come out of the Black Lives Matter (BLM) movement, which was formed by three young activist women—Alicia Garza, Patrisse Cullors, and Opal Tometi—two of whom are queer. BLM sought to ensure that women, queer, and trans people would be part of the leadership in order to provide a counterweight to the majority of liberation organizations centered around heterosexual men. Some churches have not embraced the Black Lives Matter movement because of their involvement and connection to LGBTQ liberation and affirmation. Even though the preeminent Black Liberation theologian Dr. James Cone adopted a theology of God as a God of the oppressed and sided with the poor, disenfranchised, and discriminated, the Black church has been reticent to embrace these facets of liberatory politics. It has been reluctant to pick up this theology when it comes to women making their choices for their own bodies and addressing the issue of abortion. Most of the

Black Church will not talk about liberation for same-gender-loving persons or LGBTQ people because either the pastor's theology is such that they condemn them to hell, or they are afraid that they will lose members of their congregations if the issue of affirming same-gender-loving people is brought forth to the congregation.

What could it look like to live in a world where religion and justice worked in tandem? If I just looked at it from the Christian perspective, I would say that it would look like the teaching and model of Jesus was being followed. Jesus's ministry was a ministry for those who were poor, those who were lost, left out, and discriminated against. A world where justice and religion worked in tandem would mean that religion would bring forth transformation within people, which would compel them to love and be concerned about everyone. It would mean that people would live by Dr. Martin Luther King Jr.'s words, "injustice anywhere is a threat to justice everywhere," and focused action would bring about results. Racism and White supremacy would decline. If I were to allow my imagination to grow it could affect the entire world. Famine would cease because countries that have wealth would share with poor countries. War and rumors of wars would become very difficult to transpire because transformed people would become involved in policy change and activism to make the world a better place for all.

Alas, this is not the case. Church membership and attendance is declining. We must acknowledge that even though religion is salient for Black women, and they are the most religious group in this country, there is a rise in Americans who now say they have no religious preference, and this includes all ethnicities. We do know, however, that change may start small and then build. Keeping hope alive and moving has been a characteristic of Black people and especially Black women in bringing care, health, and healing to the community.

Five

Beyond That Old Time Religion: Spirituality

Denise and her family live in a middle-class suburb of Washington, DC. When I came to interview her, she greeted me warmly with a big smile. She said she was excited to talk with me because her religion and faith were very important to her. She described herself as a spiritual person. As I entered her well-kept home, it was bright and inviting, she had pictures of her family all over her living room walls and tables I commented on how wonderful these pictures were and she then proceeded to share about each picture of her seven children and her husband. She and her twin sister grew up in foster care with an older woman who kept them involved in church, which is why she sees herself as a spiritual person now. Her husband is a minister at the church she and her entire family attend. Denise is a stay-at-home mom who does part time work as a researcher. At one point in her life, she was in the Nation of Islam, which had a great impact on her life. She still carries some of the principles of that faith with her. She reads the Bible and the Quran, which continues to guide her along with her meditation practice; she also reads Buddhist writings and other spiritual material. When asked how religion connects with her well-being, Denise said:

> Religion to me is almost like a vehicle, as Reverend Wilson states. If you don't mind, I would just love to quote him. He uses such a really great explanation of religion in that "true practice of religion should guide us in all aspects of our lives." That quote to me has just been absolutely beautiful, because to me in every aspect of my life, whether it'd be Bible or Quran, or just spiritual books that I have read, something has been able to touch me where I can use that in some form or aspect of my life.

Denise is describing how religion in some sense points her to something deeper, to spirituality. Religion has a structured set of principles and ideas that people are to adhere to, along with certain practices and rituals. Spirituality is more internal and has to do with connection and closeness to God. It provides meaning and purpose in one's life and moves one to obtain answers to difficult questions about life and relationship with the sacred. In my experience as a religious professional and mental health practitioner, many in the African American community experience religion and spirituality as one in the same. The structure of religion can point and move one to deep spirituality. Yet, when shedding light on the Spirit and what it does, this conversation can lead some in the Black Church and community to openness and others to discomfort. Engaging spirituality can move one to a transcendent dimension, where one surpasses the ordinary limits of religion.

In the worship experience in the Black Church, good preaching, instrumental music, and singing are necessary components of an effective ministry. Celebratory worship with singing, clapping, and expressive praise are components of most Black Baptist and Methodist churches. These elements can stir up emotion in individuals and help them access the sacred. However, the profound expressive experience of the Holy Spirit in the Black Holiness and Pentecostal

Church may be uncomfortable for many Black Christians. The Pentecostal movement in the United States comes from the Azusa Street Revival in Los Angeles California from 1906 to 1909. It started out as inclusive of both Black and white people under the leadership of William J. Seymour. These groups believe that to be "saved," one must undergo sanctification or holiness and "baptism of the Holy Ghost" as manifested by glossolalia or "speaking in tongues." The terminology of Holiness and Pentecostal traditions are often used interchangeably, though the Holiness tradition rejects glossolalia. Some in the Black Church fear "receiving the Holy Ghost" which can illustrate a deeper spirituality. People are afraid of what the spirit would make them do, feeling they would lose control of themselves, and that it would be undignified. There may be an emotional outpouring, manifestations that affect the whole body. People may find themselves dancing, shouting, moaning, crying, laughing, and speaking in tongues which is unintelligible to those listening, and is called being possessed by the Holy Ghost.

These traditions view speaking in tongues as biblical and find evidence for their position in the Bible. For instance, "And these signs will accompany those who believe: in my name they will drive out demons; they will speak in new tongues" (Mark 16:17, NIV); "All of them were filled with the Holy Spirit and began to speak in other tongues as the Spirit enabled them" (Acts 2:4, NIV); "When Paul placed his hands on them, the Holy Spirit came on them, and they spoke in tongues and prophesied" (Acts 19:6, NIV). According to Henry Louis Gates, in his book The Black Church: This is our Story This is our Song, the Bible interprets speaking in tongues as a gift conferred upon believers. It is this manifestation that shows authentic religious conversion and direct relationship to God.

Some in the Black church saw these manifestations, whose origins are a vestige of our African past, as embarrassing. W.E.B. Dubois found this expression of spirit possession contemptible and described it as frenzy and "trance." There has been a fear in the Black Church that these demonstrative manifestations could lead to a "reversion to heathenism." This led to a class battle which resulted in vigorous objection to any practice of charismatic religion.

My experience in the Black Church has been in the Baptist tradition. My church had a ministry of traditional Black preaching and a vibrant music ministry. There was the "card carrying" amen sister who would shout out two or three times in a service. Over the years the worship changed with some expression of dancing in the spirit, shouts of amen and waving hands. But earlier, while I was in seminary, this was not the case. At that time, I was curious about the Holy Spirit and began to visit various churches outside of my tradition. I experienced those speaking in tongues, and being slain in the spirit, with expressive praise in an African Methodist Episcopal Church. I was amazed and open to the manifestation of the spirit. Not only did I witness a move of God's Spirit, but I felt the powerful move of the spirit myself as the spirit took hold of me and showed forth power that I will never forget. I have not had any fear of this manifestation of the spirit but a knowledge that if one is open, there can be an authentic feeling that can have a depth of transformation. It is a phenomenon that is full of awe, surprise, and the unknown.

I stayed in my traditional church that underwent some transition in its worship over the years, and eventually my husband, Dr. Dennis W. Wiley, and I served as co-equal pastors for thirty-two years. Although this church has moved to more expressive worship over the years, there are some who would clearly fear such outward charismatic expression as speaking in tongues and being slain in the spirit, although from time to time it does happen. Expressive worship is sometimes seen as a class issue—worship that is practiced by those who are uneducated. This however cannot be further from the truth as there are many Black religious scholars and professionals who were raised in this tradition and speak to how it contributes positively to who they are today.

Harold Koenig and his colleagues see religion as related to community. It is structured and organized. The followers of a religion are expected to exercise certain beliefs and practices that enable individuals to have a close relationship to God. Spirituality is experienced within and is more personal. It allows one to understand questions about the meaning of life and their relationship to God.

On the other hand, African Americans historically have understood spirituality as the essence of one's entire existence, both personal and collective life: the African American experience is often tied to seeing religion and spirituality as one. As a pastor, I have found that, when African American individuals speak of their relationship with God or their faith life, they often relate this to the church and its benefits for their lives. The terms religion and spirituality are inextricably connected, and often there is a propensity to use them interchangeably.

Tynisha has found meaning in spirituality outside of traditional religion. I entered Tynisha's stairwell after she buzzed me in and went up some narrow stairs where she was waiting for me at the top landing. She was pleasant and said, "Come on in!" I greeted her, shook her hand, and entered her small apartment, which was neat. Tynisha looked a little older than her fifty stated years but was smartly dressed in makeup and long earrings. She was proud of the fact that she had a college degree.

"I have all this information and knowledge and life skills to share; however, it appears as though I'm being—is the word overlooked—if you will, for a younger person?"

When I met Tynisha, she seemed frustrated that what she perceived as ageism was preventing her from securing a job as a human service worker. She sought counseling and said she is peaceful and content in her practice of Buddhism. I sensed some bitterness as she mentioned ageism as the reason she can't get a job in her profession. She received my flyer from a local church food pantry where she receives supplemental food monthly. Tynisha shared that there are areas in spirituality that contribute to her mental well-being. She discussed the various religious modalities that have contributed to her mental well-being. She said that she likes listening to the television pastors because it appears that they are speaking directly to her. She tried reading the Bible from beginning to end but stated she couldn't do it. On occasion she will read Our Daily Bread and when she does, she stated she feels better. She admitted that she is not part of a faith community but appears to engage by reading and watching television to discover principles from various spiritual traditions. She knows the local pastor in her community, and they have talked about community issues. She talked about the history of the church and feudalism, which she said disturbs her:

> I believe in the concept of Buddhism; that's my spiritual enlightenment if you will. Actually, I believe in it . . . I enjoy the concept of it, about peace, love, harmony, can't we all get along, that type of thing. I like the idea of Gandhi, the world a

> better place, that's why I selected social work. I love the concept of Buddhism . . . and then also I'm finding that lately I bedside, what did I call it, bedside religion, I do like certain people on television like Joyce Meyer . . . I'm very diverse.

Cindy also experienced spirituality outside traditional religion. When I met Cindy at her home, she told me we would have more privacy at the local library. She listened very intently to each question and looked me directly in my eyes. She was very serious and methodical in her answers, and it appeared she had already gone through a process of soul-searching and reflection. She saw religion as different from spirituality; she did not necessarily value the rituals and wanted to move more deeply into meditation. Cindy also does not adhere to any faith practice or attend a formal gathering, but she does consider herself a Christian. When asked whether religion in any way connected with her mental well-being, she claimed to have been disappointed with church and to have found no meaning there. It is in her own personal faith and practices that she has found a deeper spirituality. She has been able to be open due to the diversity of her religious background. Asked whether religion connected to her mental well-being, she responded:

> Yes and no. I definitely have grown into more of a spiritual being in terms of just my connection with God and my growth and my journey, and the things that I've been studying, more so than religion in the sense of the rituals and the rules and the parameters. . . . For me, religion was very diverse anyway, because as a child I grew up in a Muslim background and a Christian background, and even with Christianity, was in the Baptist Church and a science background. I was exposed to a lot. Then I chose to move forth with Christianity and used to attend the church here. It just got to a point where the answers weren't coming anymore, and I needed to seek out and find more and more. I started to just grow a little bit more spiritually.

What stood out about Cindy was the appearance that she had been in an intentional process of spiritual growth. After the death of her mother from cancer, she engaged in more introspection and noted that even though her mother had admonished her to take care of herself, her mother did not do that for herself. Cindy evaluated herself and realized that she had not been valuing and caring for herself. She started to read and realize that she is a spiritual being and that her purpose in life is joy and that God is in us and thus that we do not have to search for God. Cindy went through an intentional time of self-evaluation which included her contemplation of God and how God moved in her life. She appeared to be seeking a place of spiritual well-being.

Tandy is a gay woman who is an ordained minister and belongs to an inclusive congregation that affirms the LGBTQ community. She recounted working hard in the church. She was at the church all the time, helping people, counseling them, and praying for them. She led several ministries in the church and never said no. Then there came a period when she was devastatingly hurt by her church.

> There was a position I was wanting with every fiber of my being. And when I did not get it, I went into a pretty deep depression, to the point where I needed to be seen by someone, to be seeing a therapist. But I didn't do that. Something in me realized that it was okay if I wasn't at the church all of the time. It was okay if I wasn't able to make it to where I thought I needed to be. That it was okay, that I have the right to be able to say no, to be able to take care of myself. Once I recognized that it was okay to feel the way I felt, and to do what I needed to take care of myself, I started reading theological books and the Bible and something on womanism. I started to be able to talk to people about God again just getting back to where I was before all this came about. I know mental well-being connects to religion and this is about the best I can explain it. I know that it's connected. When I am off mentally, I am off spiritually.

Tandy realized that she had been disappointed by the church and was very depressed and for a period of time did not want to go to church or talk about God or read anything religious or spiritual. It was finally when she recognized that she had to give herself permission to take care of herself that she was again able to engage in her own spirituality.

Another term that concerns the relationship between religion and mental health is spiritual well-being. Although Taylor and associates focused on religion rather than spirituality, they acknowledged that the Black Church is an organized spiritual and social community that promotes the religious, social, and psychological well-being and assimilation of individuals and families. The Black church has a history of improving the tangible lives of African Americans which suggests that spiritual matters are only one of the purposes of the Black Church. Often there is disagreement about the difference between the designations of religion and spirituality. In recent years, the term religious has almost become stigmatized with individuals seeing spirituality as a more desirable concept. However, both among Americans in general and African Americans specifically, most identify with being both religious and spiritual. My experience as a religious professional and mental health practitioner is that many in the African American community experience religion and spirituality as one in the same.

There is little consensus on the meaning of spirituality. For example, some definitions focus on an individual's belief in the existence of a sacred force that can be found in all things, a pattern of living that results from a recognition of a transcendent dimension, meaning and purpose in life, mission in life, sacredness of life, altruism, idealism, and much more. The extent to which these definitions are true for African Americans is a matter of speculation; however, Dr. Perry Halkitis and associates suggested that spirituality brings a sense of health and psychological well-being to African Americans.

When coping with all that can happen in our day-to-day lives, using religious resources may help individuals adjust their thinking and feeling so that their mental and spiritual health is improved. On the other hand, spiritual well-being is an inner sense that assists in dealing with life's struggles, and gives one a sense of purpose and meaning, encompassing the individual's integrity, beliefs, and habits.

The spiritual well-being (SWB) scale is a comprehensive measure of an individual's perception of their overall well-being. SWB is not a psychological measurement. It combines religious well-being (RWB), which refers to a sense of contentment and inner peace that comes from religious beliefs and practices, with existential well-being (EWB), which refers to a sense of fulfillment and satisfaction with life that comes from finding meaning and purpose. It involves feeling connected to something greater than oneself.

It is known that a core value of African American women is spirituality. In examining both the coping skills and spiritual well-being using the Brief R-Cope measure of religious coping scale, Natalie Arnette and her colleagues assessed African American women impacted by domestic violence. Survivors have pointed to spirituality as being meaningful to them. Spiritual well-being refers not only to having meaning in one's life, but also relationship with God.

However, without interventions or resources in the face of domestic violence, a relationship with God doesn't always lead to high levels of spiritual well-being. Tricia Bent-Goodley and her colleagues note that partner abuse tends to be more violent among African Americans than any other ethnic group. When interventions such as support services and groups, education, protected environments, and counseling services are used along with spirituality, there appeared to be positive indicators for psychological well-being.

Clinicians who work with traumatized African American women may ask them about the importance of religion and spirituality in their lives. Many clients want their spiritual issues addressed, which in turn can aid them in their coping skills and spiritual well-being. Counselors can help with their religious coping by encouraging religious involvement and allowing them to share their religious and spiritual struggles and apprehensions in their treatment.

Religious coping and spiritual well-being have some similarities. Both refer to a sense of well-being with individuals and bring comfort and a sense of closeness to God which allows for intimacy with others. Both religious coping and spiritual well-being imply a person's recognition of a transcendent God. With religious coping and with spiritual well-being, individuals can find meaning in their lives.

While there are similarities between religious coping and spiritual well-being, there are also differences. Whereas religious coping allows an individual to solve problems, that is not necessarily the desired outcome with spiritual well-being. When things appear to be unmanageable in a person's life, religious coping can help. Spiritual well-being is relevant both in situations of calm and chaos. Neither religious coping nor spiritual well-being require the use of religious resources such as prayer, church participation, or counseling by clergy; prayer however, is a highly used resource for spiritual well-being. Religious coping can be understood as a process, while spiritual well-being can be seen as a state of being. Spiritual well-being is personal, subjective, and internal, whereas religious coping can be both internal and external.

Although Donelda Cook and I found that African Americans frequently make no differentiation between one's spirituality, identity, or religion, my study demonstrated varied understandings and approaches to the term religion, as each woman had her own assessment of what this term meant to her. No prior definitions or interpretations of the terms for religion or mental well-being were given to the women in this study.

Some women discussed their experience with church when asked how religion connected with their mental well-being. Church appeared to be central in many of these women's lives. They focused on the positive relationships in the church, the ability to serve and volunteer, in addition to what they learned from their pastor. In some sense, they showed a belief that the church helped them in their overall lives more than other resources in the community. The church provided prayer, comfort, and support, and helped women become close to God.

Another focus of the interviews was God and women's relationship with God. These women shared of a connection with God that changed them and healed them. They felt supported and grounded by God. Some spoke of religious writings pointing them to God and helping them to feel spiritually connected with increased faith and a feeling of hope and strength. They also described a sense of purpose and self-awareness, as women also talked about being in communication with God.

Other participants emphasized their faith. This had to do with an intense belief that there was something within them that allowed them to believe and hold onto as real in their lives. This something within was able to guide and assist and keep them in times of extreme difficulty even in the face of situations that appeared to be hopeless. They expressed a certainty that it was a faith within them that "brought them through" and empowered them. A couple of the women also expressed their doubts, wondering whether they had been helped by a higher power, assisted by their prayers, or whether it was just circumstance. Nevertheless, faith was clearly the center of what religion was for them.

Spirituality was a term chosen by women who appeared to have been introduced to several religious ideologies and or institutions and chose not to reject any, but to take out of these traditions what was helpful for them. They indeed did separate spirituality from religion and saw spirituality as something to be desired beyond religiosity. They saw themselves as spiritual beings; furthermore, some of them used meditation and what sounded like mindfulness practice even though they were not necessarily familiar with this term. As Tynisha explained: "I love the concept of Buddhism . . . I'm very diverse . . . Buddhism has helped me to be, to have a peace of mind and to realize that it's not me most of the time." Although admitting to enjoying watching Christian evangelists on the television, when asked what is helpful for her religiously, Tynisha responded "the practices," referring to Buddhist practice.

Cindy stated that when she was overwhelmed, her spiritual practice was to breathe and meditate.

> I guess in my studies and a lot of the pieces that I read, I've adopted a lot of other meditations that are out there. So, I try to do well; I know that first and foremost that I just need to stop when I'm feeling overwhelmed. I need to take that time to just kind of go general and just bring it back and not be caught up into the details. I just do some deep breathing, and just trying to just say, yes, because I know all things will work out for me, but not in the middle of the details and the panic. Then in terms of meditating, sometimes it's an active meditation and sometimes it's just to myself in solace. I've learned how to have meditations in the sense of just almost kind of using affirmations and finding something peaceful to focus on, or finding a thought to focus on, a positive thought that can divert my attention away from whatever seems to be that issue.

Although Denise saw church as very important to her and talked about being raised in the church, meditation as a construct different from prayer is what helped her keep mental well-being:

> I don't read scripture every day, but what I will say is that when I know I need to take breaks, I will just quietly sit, and I may meditate. When my children were growing up, I had a ritual, a daily ritual where they would take a nap, or they would have to be quiet for a good hour, because they knew that mommy was downstairs meditating. The peace of mind to know that bringing them up, they would have to oblige by that, unless someone was hurt, physically hurt, you don't bother mommy

during this time. It was more so my eldest daughter and my eldest twin sons, they were the ones who would experience that, that mommy is meditating. Even if they come into the house now and if they come in my room and they see me just sitting very quietly, oh mommy is meditating. Just don't bother her at this point in time.

Valencia admitted to having experience with meditation, but because it was outside her tradition in the church, she kept it to herself and became somewhat wary of it.

Yeah, a young man, he taught me that you should learn how to meditate, just try to learn how to go outside your body. He gave me these powerful books to read about the mind, and I read them, and I started trying to meditate. I'd go into meditation just like I'm asleep and then I think of God. I always want to meet him and what I would definitely like; I could feel him on me and stuff. I went, sat in a chair and closed my eyes and I just talked to him and just relaxed and just let my body float. It seemed like I left my body. When I left my body, I felt like I was in heaven. I just felt like I'd seen Jesus. When I came back, it was like a scary and good thing too, because it felt good up there but to come back and I woke up like wow that was really deep. I said I don't know if I'm ready for that much yet.

In some of the research on African Americans and religion, meditation and prayer have been understood as the same construct, but some scholars perceive meditation as a distinct construct separate from prayer that has to do with concentrated contemplation, focused breathing, stillness, quiet, and reflection. The General Social Survey of the United States noted that two out of three African Americans participate in meditation and slightly more than fifty percent of all African Americans meditate once a week. In addition, a stress reduction program found that transcendental meditation considerably decreased the combined finality of heart attacks, stroke, and mortality in African American patients with coronary heart disease.

The aforementioned studies may be surprising to many African Americans who are interested in religion, because meditation is not a general practice of the church even though their church members are meditating. Indeed, some churches warn parishioners against practices of East Asian origins such as meditation and yoga. Based upon my experience as clergy within the Black church tradition in the United States, which is often seen as quite conservative, meditation and yoga are sometimes received with outright rejection and skepticism. At the same time, churches that have a more progressive theology are open to these modalities.

Although religion and spirituality are often considered one and the same by African Americans, I do see them as different constructs. One can be religious without being spiritual, and one can be spiritual without being religious. This can be confusing sometimes because sometimes the terms religion and spirituality are used interchangeably.

Religion is carried out in faith communities such as churches, mosques, and temples, which require persons to adhere to certain expectations. An individual could go through the motions of following the expectations of the religious community without any internal transformation or change. Spirituality is a connection to the transcendent. It signifies going beyond one's ordinary physical understanding and experiencing a supernatural, boundless, and supreme God or the sacred. The transcendent is that which is outside of the self, and yet also within the self. Spirituality is connected to the mystical and to religion but extends beyond organized religion. Spirituality embraces a quest for the transcendent and encountering the transcendent. It is a progressive process that may move one to question one's beliefs or to embrace a new belief. Belief can lead to devout commitment and ultimately, submission.

Spirituality can impact individuals such that they not only feel close to the sacred but feel better about themselves. There is an inner transformation in which peace and a new positive direction in life may be found. Spirituality can increase the quality of relationships, deepen values, and give a sense of purpose in life. One may ask deep questions regarding issues such as suffering or death, and may feel a sense of compassion and empathy to others. As noted earlier, some manifestations of the spirit such as speaking in tongues, dancing, and shouting, running, and bodily movements make people uncomfortable, resulting in some faith traditions feeling negative about overt spirituality. Although in a worshipping context, these "manifestations of the spirit" appear to be authentic, some may focus on the outward showing of the spirit with no inner transformation. Some religious traditions practice overt prayers and condemnation of those they believe need to be delivered from demons, which can be harmful, especially for people of marginalized identities or people with drug dependencies. These outward expressions of spirituality differ greatly from the inner quest for spiritual growth.

It is true that there can sometimes be negative experiences with spirituality and church. Adverse interaction among church members along with church conflict can make some resistant to spirituality; however, those who participate in religion are often moved to a deeper level of spirituality. They have better health outcomes than those who don't. Using religious resources such as prayer, reading religious materials, meditation, and attending religious programming has been helpful for Black women. Prayer has been an effective coping mechanism and the ability to experience church members as a source of social support has been uplifting and beneficial.

As I have noted, it was spirituality as an adult that I experienced before religion. Whether it is connected to organized religion or not, spirituality can help Black women as oppressed people to navigate the difficulties in life such as systemic racism, sexism, discrimination in the workplace, and help them to cope with their day-to-day difficulties. Just because some Black women don't go to church does not mean that they don't have a relationship with a higher power. Spirituality can give women a sense of joy and peace and allow them to negotiate how to live their lives in a mentally healthy way. More and more women are involved in mindfulness meditation and transcendental meditation which helps to bring healthy minds and wholeness. Reading scripture, praying, and reading positive material for Black women stand alongside yoga as beneficial practices.

Finding a faith community that is progressive and positive toward women can be something that can be very helpful in Black women's lives. Finding a good community of faith that fits you is an undertaking. Just like you really must assess and evaluate finding a partner in your life, you must do the same thing with a worshiping community. Using resources that fit you in the church can aid and deepen your spirituality; if one church does not fit you, there is another not too far away that will fit you well, knowing that no church is perfect. You have to take your responsibility in your own spiritual growth.

Six

When Faith Fails

While some Black women find strength in spirituality, others feel they have been let down by the church and become ambivalent toward religion. I met Linda in her home. She is an attractive 43-year-old woman who walks with a slight limp because she has a prosthetic leg. She had received my flyer from a friend and appeared to be somewhat nervous in the beginning but as we started talking, she appeared more relaxed. She lives with her husband. He was very gracious and pleasant, and she appeared to be very comfortable introducing the two of us. As Linda loosened up, she shared what she thought about religion.

"I think it's a good thing [religion], but dependent upon what the issue is, I think that some type of counseling probably can also coincide with their faith as well." Linda works in the human service field, and she appears ambivalent regarding religion; however, she states she does pray and every now and then will go to church.

Linda has some uncertainty about the church, and even whether God is real. On the one hand, she states that she prays but appears unsure about whether it is working for her. She says after she prays things usually do turn out to be ok, but there is some skepticism in her voice and demeanor. She stated, "A lot of people always encouraged me to pray about whatever it is I may be going through . . . usually I do that, and things do turn out to be okay." In her sharing, it appeared that she really wasn't sure whether prayer had anything to do with the situation turning out to be okay or not. Linda sees herself as an introvert. She goes to a church sometimes because she finds the church authentic. However, she still has some discomfort regarding expressive praise in worship. She says she feels better when she goes to church, even though she has underlying questions as to whether there is a God. It appears that she doesn't know if she really wants to believe and her doubts overwhelm her. She has given no indication as to where these feelings come from. When I have met other Black women who have had this sense of ambivalence, it has had to do with trauma they have experienced, and sometimes the trauma was in some way connected to the church. Or perhaps there is a feeling that the church is hypocritical and judgmental. Some people do not like the culture of faith communities, which can be exclusive and even strange to those experiencing the practices for the first time. Rituals can appear to be meaningless and difficult to understand. At the same time, people may also see some positive value in them.

Religious ambivalence is a state of having simultaneous conflicting reactions, beliefs, or feelings towards religion and the religious experience. Religious ambivalence can be inspired by a variety of factors, including individual experiences, exposure to different religious beliefs, questioning of religious teachings and practices, and cultural and societal influences. Conflicting beliefs about religion or facets of it may cause an individual to waver between different concepts and feel doubtful about their beliefs. Some people, such as Linda, may question the notion of God or the authenticity of various religious doctrines or observances. As I mentioned, trauma or challenging experiences such as the loss of a loved one can cause persons to question their faith or struggle with their religious beliefs.

Linda's ambivalence was clear as she talked about God and about the church. She is a clinician who appears to be skeptical about her clients' dependence on their faith. She has also struggled with her own depression and has been on medication and in counseling: "When I think about what people say, how they just rely on God to get them through certain things. Sometimes I'm thinking about like is there really a God?" Linda further indicated that sometimes religion felt uncomfortable for her: "Sometimes it does, even when I go to church, sometimes it does. I don't know why that is, but sometimes it does. Then sometimes I'll watch other people and just see how they are just comfortable enough to like praise him and all that, I'm just not in that space yet."

Linda appeared to have more faith in counseling than in religion or belief:

> **Most people will try to seek some type of counseling or what have you, but a lot of the clients that I have come across and worked with, they really just rely on their faith to get through whatever obstacles it is that they're going through. I think that I've seen that more amongst African Americans than any other people. I think that some type of counseling probably can also coincide with their faith as well. This is just my opinion; I don't think that one should just rely on their faith.**

Black clinicians know that religion and spirituality are core values of the African American community, as many have come out of these religious traditions themselves. Discerning a woman's experience with and assessment of religion can be helpful for clinicians, who can not only use therapeutic methods, but give clients permission to talk about their faith, whether it be strong or ambivalent. Understanding whether the client has experienced trauma related to religion and establishing trust between client and clinician can help clients talk about how this trauma affected them and what it means to them. Clinicians can give a more holistic view to women by informing them that there are many religious traditions and cultures even in Christianity, and that not all Christian experiences and beliefs are the same. Providing a safe space for women to talk can allow women to move from ambivalence to a place that is more grounded and peaceful. It can be detrimental for women when clinicians refuse to discuss their religious ambivalence. Some may tell women to talk to their pastors about their concerns. It is possible to understand those with religious ambivalence better if we listen intently to them and do not judge them. Clinicians should respect their beliefs even if they do not agree with them. They may ask questions to get a better understanding and avoid making assumptions about their beliefs or experiences. But they can also offer support and resources that can help the individual who is struggling with their beliefs or experiences to help them direct their religious ambivalence in a healthy manner. I believe that clinicians should be able to meet individuals where they are by addressing spiritual issues if it is called for. If not addressed in the counseling room, this can be something that continues to be unsettling for women, preventing them from moving towards wholeness.

There are some women whose trauma is directly connected to a pastor, elder, deacon, steward, or leader in the church. These women may have been sexually assaulted by a pastor or leader in the church. This experience can cause a great deal of trauma so that when women find themselves in a faith institution, religious setting, or church, they can be triggered. This means they might re-experience symptoms of the trauma which can manifest itself as intense emotional distress. Clinicians who give trauma-informed care make sure that trust is developed between the clinician and the woman, that they are safe, they can make their own choices, and collaboratively they can work together to focus on strengths and move towards individual empowerment. They take care not to retraumatize. Social workers and mental health providers should have the ability to meet individuals where they are with a compassionate, empathetic, and non-critical approach. It does not matter whether a clinician has a religious background themselves or not. As clinicians, they should be able to "cross the cultures," using the strengths of the individual and helping them build on these strengths. Working with individuals who have experienced multiple traumas can be particularly challenging, requiring significant patience and understanding. Yasmin is one who has some ambivalence regarding structured religion.

Yasmin is a 25-year-old African American woman of short stature with beautiful hair and eyes. She is currently working on her third graduate degree, a doctorate in education. She is active in her sorority and is an ordained minister in her church. She appears younger than her stated years and speaks hurriedly and appears to be thinking as she is talking. What stood out about her was she took each question I asked her very seriously and pondered the question as she spoke. She was living with a friend temporarily in a nice neighborhood and the home was very spacious. Although we both had ample space to sit, she stood the entire time, taking in every question and providing detailed responses.

Although most of the women interviewed expressed positive feelings about religion, that is not the case for a few. Yasmin explained that she felt both good and bad about religion at times. This ambivalence has had to do with how she has negatively experienced the Black Church, which she feels is judgmental and has not always been a place that would meet her where she is. Yasmin has struggled with depression and felt that the church was not a safe place to reveal this. She felt she would be criticized that she did not pray enough or have enough faith if she revealed her depression. Growing up in the Black church, Yasmin experienced the church family as being judgmental if someone revealed that they were depressed. This made her feel bad about herself, thinking she did not have enough faith, or did not pray enough as some of the members of her church had counseled others. When I asked Yasmin how religion made her feel about herself, she answered:

> Sometimes good, sometimes like the scum of the earth. As silent as some black homes can be about mental health and mental well-being, I feel like the church can be equally silent. I found myself in this conflict . . . like can I really say that I'm a believer if I get sad, if I get depressed, if I'm confronting this thing. I feel like what ends up happening sometimes is you just kind of pretend that what you feel like isn't real. It's like oh but I believe, so it's just gone, and I'm just healed, but you did no work. It's like no, it's not gone, because you didn't deal with it. I feel like in some ways like religion almost does a disservice.

It is true that historically, Black women have faced discrimination and marginalization in the church, which at times can feel like an unsafe space for them. Some Black churches certainly maintain an understanding and theology that holds that men should be in charge, that women cannot teach men, and that women must obey their husbands. Misogyny exists in the patriarchal nature of many

Black churches, which leads to Black women feeling that they are treated unfairly and their voices not heard. This plays into the negative stigma around church and religion. In my counseling practice, I have come upon several women who have experienced gender-based violence in the church including sexual assault. Sometimes pastors have not supported women who have reported domestic violence in the home. They have been told to obey their husbands. These women have often not received the support they needed to heal and recover from this trauma. I am careful to say that of course this is not all Black churches. Many pastors are acutely aware of the oppression of Black women and move to have ministries that are empowering of them, encouraging leadership from the pulpit to the pew.

One problem that has not been addressed in many Black churches, however, is homophobia. The Black Church is known for its anti-LGBTQ views, which has made it an unsafe place for Black women who identify as LGBTQ or same-gender-loving. This has defined Tandy's experience. She notes that religion can so often be used as a weapon, and she has to be careful of the places she puts herself in as a gay woman:

> When I was in seminary one of my preaching professors took us to his church to preach, to do our sermons. And everyone who preached that night preached a sermon of hate, very homophobic. It was horrible. And to the point where one of the teaching aids leaned over to me and asked me if I was okay. I mean it was "The Black Church experience." Folks were standing up shouting, she asked me if I was okay and I said no. She asked if I wanted to leave and I said no, they are not going to run me out of here. That has been the most uncomfortable I've ever been. And the most afraid I've ever been in the church. The professor invited his congregation and they were there too. I refuse to be run out of the church. But I sat there through 4 or 5 sermons condemning me to hell.

Tandy said that it was her faith in God and her spiritual connection that got her through this difficult time.

Another area that women have felt unsafe about is revealing their own bouts with depression. Like Yasmin, some have felt that if you feel depressed, then you have a lack of faith or weak faith. This harmful misconception can cause some to feel guilty or ashamed about their depression. What we know is ongoing depression is a medical condition that is in no way related to the strength of one's faith. Some may feel that faith can cure depression and while faith is a good coping mechanism and can provide strength and support, it is important to acknowledge that depression is a mental health condition that often requires professional treatment such as counseling and medication.

There are also those in the church that think that prayer is effective and is enough to treat depression. While prayer is a helpful coping resource and tool for depression, it cannot replace evidenced-based treatments such as therapy and medication. Another misconception is that people of faith cannot experience depression. What we know is that anyone can experience depression regardless of their beliefs or religion. Many churches now have counseling ministries with licensed professionals who provide therapy and counseling. They may provide seminars and Bible studies on depression. In the biblical text there are many instances of those who suffer from depression. David was distressed and depressed and dealt with deep despair over the loss of his sons; Elijah was discouraged, tired and afraid as he ran from the threats of Jezebel; Job experienced great loss and devastation and exclaimed "Why did I not perish at birth, and die as I came from the womb?" Moses was depressed over the sin of his people's betrayal.

Depression is a human experience. In the biblical text King David in Psalms 42 expressed feelings of despair and sadness and writes "Why my soul are you so downcast, why so disturbed within me?" The prophet Elijah experienced deep sadness and even wished for death in 1 Kings 19. Faithful people can struggle with depression, and it is part of the human experience. Clinical depression however, is a mental health condition characterized by persistent feelings of sadness, hopelessness, and a loss of interest or pleasure in activities. It is different from normal sadness or grief, as it can significantly impact a person's daily functioning and quality of life.

Depression can have a plethora of symptoms and vary from person to person. There can be symptoms such as persistent sadness and anxiety, and feelings of hopelessness, worthlessness, or helplessness. Loss of interest in the things that used to bring one joy and lack of energy or fatigue along with difficulty sleeping or oversleeping can be present. Appetite and weight changes along with difficulty focusing or concentrating, and restlessness or irritability are signs and symptoms. Physical symptoms can also show up such as headaches, digestive problems, pain, and thoughts of death or suicide. As we contemplate these symptoms of depression, we know that there can be serious consequences; that is why it is so important to seek mental health care to those who are suffering with this disorder. However, there are those who may say that God has "healed" them from depression or mental illness. Is it possible for there to be a miraculous healing of depression and other mental health conditions? There are those who have claimed to be supernaturally healed and those who say they have witnessed such a healing. If God wants to heal someone miraculously then God certainly has the right and the ability to do so. We do have to pay attention however that "miraculous healing" is often subjective and could mean different things to different people. It is important to think critically and to note that a variety of factors could be involved such as a placebo effect, psychosomatic symptoms, and a natural recovery process. While faith and spirituality can be significant sources of comfort and support in the face of depression and mental health challenges, it is important to prioritize professional treatment and support to ensure the best possible outcomes for individuals struggling with depression and other mental health conditions.

The fact of the matter is, coping with depression and embracing faith is a challenging process; there is no 'one size fits all" solution. There are some things that can help. Seek a mental health professional who can provide tools and strategies to help manage the symptoms of depression. Pastoral psychotherapists are mental health professionals who have expertise in spirituality and can also provide therapeutic religious and spiritual resources. Talking to a trusted spiritual leader can provide guidance as you navigate your spiritual journey. Practicing self-care is important, taking care of body mind and spirit. This means eating well, getting enough sleep, engaging in regular exercise, and participating in activities that bring you joy. Then, focus on gratitude. Practicing gratitude every day can help to shift your focus away from negative thoughts and feelings. You can make a list of things you are grateful for each day. Meditation and prayer can bring forth a sense of peace and calm and change your outlook, as well as the practice of journaling. Also support groups and discipleship groups can be very helpful. They can be safe spaces where individuals are able to hear others who struggle with the same issues and know that they are not alone. They can be a space of accountability where members connect in relationship to one another and hold each other accountable for what they said they would do to move forward and heal. I have seen people experience encouragement and strength in these groups where they have been able to face what they feared or move from their pain and become more whole as people. Individuals may have to try different practices until they find what works for them. Everyone's journey is different. It is important to be patient and compassionate with yourself as you navigate this process.

Both Linda and Yasmin have a sense of unsureness. Linda is not sure that someone should lean totally into their faith when they are going through "whatever obstacles" they endure. She alludes to the notion that professional counseling and mental health care is needed. Yasmin feels you can't trust the church in sharing about your depression or struggles because the church is judgmental, and religion does a disservice by indicating in some way that religion alone is sufficient. It appears that religious ambivalence in Black women can sometimes lead them to rely on clinical health rather than faith. Mental health services using evidence-based practices are clearly needed to combat the depression, trauma, and oppression that many Black women experience. My contention is that you must meet women where they are. If strong faith is a tool that is important for these women, then along with mental health modalities, using religious resources that help women to cope such as prayer, meditation and even corporate worship can be very helpful. Because religion and spirituality are core values in the African American community, using religious resources within the context of the therapeutic relationship between therapist and client can be very beneficial for the individual who holds these values. Black women need to care for body, mind, and spirit. For example, practicing yoga benefits the body, mind, and spirit using mindfulness meditation to improve overall sense of well-being. Adding psychotherapy, also known as talk therapy or counseling, when one is struggling with depression or other mental health disorders, helps individuals to better understand their thoughts, feelings, and behaviors which can lead to increased self-awareness. Therapy can help one with coping skills, enhance problem solving, and can be an effective treatment for balance and fulfillment in their lives.

As a Black woman who is a pastoral psychotherapist and a social worker, I try to find out what has helped women in the past when they have been having trouble. If they say that God, or reading the Bible, or prayer has been helpful, I will ask them whether it might be helpful to them to use any of these resources in our sessions together. I will then incorporate these religious resources into the Psychodynamic, Cognitive Behavioral Therapy, Trauma focused Therapy, Dialectical Behavioral Therapy, or whatever modality I am using. If religion or spirituality is not part of the value system of an individual or they do not want to use these resources, I will then just proceed with my assessment and therapeutic intervention. I am very aware and must keep in mind that some women's experience of religion has them feeling ambivalent or there has been something traumatic that has happened to them within the church, with a church leader, or around religious people. These experiences make it very difficult for women to connect with faith.

Seven

Empowerment

Kelly is a 46-year-old social worker who looks much younger than her years. She works at an agency where she is in a school, working with children and families. She is an ordained minister and serves as the youth pastor at her church. Kelly takes her ministry seriously bringing new opportunities to youth and meeting them where they are. She has been passionately working with children and youth for many years. She has an engaging smile, beautiful medium brown skin, and piercing brown eyes. She is very attractive and often wears Afrocentric attire and jewelry and wears her hair in locks. She still lives in the urban community that she grew up in, which she says was long her dream. Her community is in the most densely populated area of the city and has the largest number of children and youth. It also has the highest crime rate and the lowest number of young people graduating with a high school diploma. She is single and has a busy life with her family, which consists of her father, a brother, and a sister. Her mother died some years ago. She had a heavy influence on Kelly as she was also a social worker who was conscientious, committed, and dedicated to her work and had a significant impact in the community. Kelly has her own community ministry working with teenage girls. Several of the young girls she has aided went with her on a college tour and ultimately attend college. Her ministry not only kept the girls off the street but helped them boost their self-esteem. Some experienced traumas in the home and community and this ministry became a safe haven for them.

Kelly was interviewed in her home, which she owns. It is a row house that is decorated very smartly. Her father owns two apartment buildings on the street she lives on, and each of her family members (father and two siblings) own their own home on the street. Kelly appeared to be very confident and excited to participate in the interview. She seemed to be someone that I might like to be friends with. She had a lot of energy and what she characterized as a calling to make things better for those living in the community where she lived and worked.

Kelly is a Kellogg Fellow. The William Keith Kellogg Foundation gives grants to individuals and organizations that help vulnerable children. Kelly was working with the racial equity and healing cohort at the time of her interview. Kelly lived around, worked with, and went to church with young people whose community did not have the resources to give them a healthy and abundant life. She wanted to do something for young people and their families in a system of poverty and oppression. She saw obstacles to opportunity and education. She knew that these systemic issues endangered self-esteem and reinforced problematic reactions in individuals, families, and communities.

As Kelly was unmarried, she filled her life with purpose. Being in relationship with young people and their families gave her joy. Her deep faith had her also trying to connect young people and their families to God and to the church. Several of the families she brought to her church first connected with the church's food pantry. When they took a risk to come to worship, they found that it was a welcoming and inclusive space. Kelly's relationship building helped those who are often forgotten. As Kelly had this outlook in life, she felt fulfilled and empowered. She used her faith for her own sense of empowerment and liberation.

As I talked with Kelly, it became apparent to me that her thinking was closely in line with the principles and beliefs of womanist theology. As noted, womanist theology considers the connections between gender, race, racism, sexism, and power. Womanist theology, which is spiritualized, observes how oppressive systems have shaped the lives of African American women. It puts forward a vision of religion that enables women to use it for their empowerment and liberation. Since womanist theology is a spiritual construct, this spirituality in both womanism and religion can engender strength and fortitude in women to continue forward in their lives, despite their struggle, Women seek a positive quality of life, often in the face of an oppressive society that blocks them from the freedom and well-being they desire.

Those who are oppressed and in need of support are also those who band together to attain more power. Women, especially African American women, want to attain more power in both their personal and public lives. The women in my study overwhelmingly felt positive about their view of religion, feeling that religion improved their mental well-being. Many spoke of feeling confident. They spoke of feeling special and important to God. This feeling that their lives were better for their encounter with religion intersects directly with empowerment.

With respect to empowerment theory, Barbara Solomon argued that discrimination, especially the intersection of racism and sexism, may leave women paralyzed without the ability to cope with internal frustrations and struggles, due to the power blocks of daily life. This powerlessness contributes to poor health, both physically and emotionally, in the lives of women. Religion can become a support system that can empower and move African American women towards positive action.

Considering religion as a support that engenders mental well-being in women does not entail ignoring the inequities and struggles in the lives of the women in my study. Although some of the women are highly educated, they nevertheless have challenges in their lives. Some are burdened with mental illness, poverty, unemployment, and lack of education. Often these factors are due to the systemic oppression that continues to exist in our society.

I think of how it impacts the Black community even from within. In Zora Neale Hurston's novel Their Eyes Were Watching God, Nanny Crawford says, "So de white man throw down de load and tell the [Black] man tuh pick it up. He pick it up because he have to, but he don't tote it. He hand it to his women folks." This quote depicts how Black women have traditionally been situated at the lowest point in American social hierarchy. Sojourner Truth's admonition that she expects to be treated just as well as any white woman fell on deaf ears, as she says, "I have borne thirteen children, and seen most all sold off to slavery, and when I cried out with my mother's grief, none but Jesus heard me! And ain't I a woman?" If there is to be equality in these United States of America, Black women have a voice and move to effective action. In recent times, there appears to be a move away from progressive values that uphold justice and equality for marginalized individuals. Instead, a growing number of people are beginning to subscribe to conservative beliefs that seem to support racism and white supremacy. This shift presents an alarming pattern, which threatens to promote bigotry and social injustices that have long plagued our society. The challenge, therefore, lies in creating a balance that respects people of all races, religions, and cultures, while enabling us to move forward, united as a community. In 2015, a landmark ruling was made by the United States Supreme Court that granted marriage equality across the nation, allowing same-sex couples the right to marry in all 50 states. However, a few years earlier, the Supreme Court also invalidated key provisions of the 1965 Voting Rights Act, which was designed to protect the voting rights of minorities and prevent discriminatory practices at the polls. This decision ultimately weakened the protections against voter discrimination and allowed certain states to implement voter ID laws and redistricting plans that disenfranchised minority communities. Since this time, the John R. Lewis Voting Right Advancement Act has failed in the Congress, although it continues to be reintroduced

Despite overt discrimination against Black people that has become the law of the land, Black women have often used these injustices as a springboard to their activism. Indeed, Black women have been the driving force of social justice movements throughout American history. They have been the Democratic Party's most reliable and devoted voting bloc and helped to deliver the election for President Joe Biden in 2020. In keeping with the womanist spirit, it is my belief that Black women's social and political engagement brings wholeness for the entire community, which encompasses empowerment, inclusivity, social change, liberation, and well-being. Black women attaining more power in the Black community is important to me because it brings a positive spirit and diversity into the mainstream and brings the opportunity for positive interrelations through dialogue and connection.

I have come to a place where I am very comfortable in my relationship with God, understanding finally that God loves me and wants the best for me. That wasn't always the case. When my first husband was committing adultery and drinking too much, I felt depressed and unworthy. It was only when I got enough courage through prayer and supportive people around me that I was able to leave and file for divorce. It was then that I started to feel more self-assured. My first husband and I had gone to counseling, and I even took him to the preacher, but it was clear that he was unwilling to change his lifestyle. I remember going over and over in my mind that I had taken a vow to be with this person in sickness and in health. I said, "Maybe he is sick" and I need to just keep praying for him. At some point, "something came to me" saying that perhaps God did not want me to be with this person, endure this adversity; that perhaps I deserved better. Because of my involvement in the church and spiritual resources like the Bible, prayer, meditation, and attending church, I became empowered to see myself differently and understand that God wanted something better for me. It was as if I experienced the phrase that Black preachers have used, and is often in gospel songs, "God picked me up, turned me around, and placed my feet on solid ground." This meant that I found authentic strength and stability in God's, presence, God's action, and God's guidance and support.

As we consider the attainment of more power for Black women, some of the interviews in this book demonstrate that religion can engender confidence in some women. I myself felt this pull by the Spirit of God to draw closer and to live my life and purpose for God. It was then that I connected with the church, which enabled me to encounter others who also were serious about their faith. As I worked in the mental health field, I encountered mentally ill adults and children and came to see them as people who belonged to God. I felt compelled to ensure that they received the best possible treatment, and part of my responsibility was to improve the quality of their lives. It was in this work that I became confident in my relationship with God and my purpose of helping people to grow and develop and to be comfortable with themselves and their relationships. In addition, it was in my own spiritual growth and development that I became more confident in myself and divorced my first husband and now have been married to a wonderful man for many years.

Over many years of seeing a diversity of Black women in counseling and therapy, I have experienced histories that prompt them to feel unworthy, afraid, and stuck. This leads them to develop behaviors that are unhealthy and unproductive, and they don't feel good about themselves. It is in our work together that women have been able to understand that their conditions had often come about through no fault of their own. In our work together, they developed new ways of thinking and put away the erroneous thoughts that had them feeling badly, often about themselves, and replaced those thoughts with the truth about themselves. When I asked women what were some strengths that had helped them in the past in difficulty, many spoke of God. Some were open to talking about God and admitted feeling that God was blaming them or not supportive or helpful to them. We often unearthed the fact that they may have had an idolatrous God. For example, if they had neglectful parents, they may have seen God as one who sits high, looks low, and does nothing. If they had a very critical or even abusive parent or caretaker, they may have seen God as highly critical and sometimes even abusive. Our work included discussing who the true God really was for them. It was in our collaboration that I experienced women blossoming, becoming more confident in themselves, and taking risks to improve the quality of their lives.

Although I do not remember living my life without the felt presence of God, I do remember being depressed thinking that this was just the way life was supposed to be. I knew God was present, but in my life, it felt like God did nothing. It was when I was in my deepest despair that I finally cried out to God to help me. I was able finally to see the truth and reality of things, which gave me the courage to leave that situation, seek a divorce, and then find a church. I remember feeling so sad and depressed. I remember having such unhappiness. Today that seems like another life. Yes, I still do have some difficulties in my life, but I have a connection to God that keeps me grounded. I am not perfect, but I do feel good about me. I have a sense of joy and write in my journal every day three things I am grateful for. My mistakes are mistakes; I don't have to belittle myself for them. I feel like a child of God with a history of some trauma and addictions in my family and self-worth issues that have been transformed. It feels as if God has called me "out of the darkness into [God's] marvelous light" (1 Peter 2:9 NRSV).

Becky is someone else who has experienced depression and undergone some trauma in her life. She described how she felt good despite some day-to-day challenges. Becky has a history of physical and sexual abuse, and, when she struggles with bouts of depression, she uses her faith to push her to do whatever it is she feels she has to.

> How does it [religion] make me feel about myself? I feel great. I feel great, yes, I do. I have my up and down days. I even have days of, you know, what I don't even feel like talking to God today, I don't feel like praying today. Then I would say wait a minute that's the enemy. He is trying to get me, you know what I'm saying? Because that's his job to kill, steal, and destroy, and he is trying to sift me like a grain of wheat but, no, I got a plan, God has the plan for me, and I have some work I have to do. I'm going to have to tell myself that sometimes to get myself a bottle of funk or sometimes it takes a situation to put your back up against the wall where you have no one to call on but God.

Becky has found that God is a resource when your back is up against the wall and you have no one else to call upon. Historically, Black women have had to deal with the intersections of adversity in its many configurations. These have included racial and gender discrimination, unequal access to education and employment opportunities, lower pay and wealth accumulation, lack of healthcare access amid stereotypes, and bias in media and society. All these issues affect Black women in addition to their own personal traumas and history. Many Black women have faced these challenges and felt they had no one to call on but Jesus. These encounters with adversity can lead to higher levels of poverty, lower rates of home ownership and business ownership, and higher rates of maternal and infant mortality. In the midst of such oppression, Becky uses her faith to "push" herself to do whatever she feels she must do. Many Black women use faith as a source of strength and empowerment in their lives. It can inspire Black women to pursue their goals for themselves, their children, and their communities, even in the face of obstacles and challenges. Using their faith in this manner allows Black women to get in touch with their own internal power and resilience. This faith can be a formidable tool for empowerment.

On the other hand, this notion of the "strong Black woman" sometimes moves women to remain strong at all costs. Black women are expected to uphold their strength in the face of even the most intense pain or fear. Unfortunately, expressing their emotions is often discouraged as it may be perceived as a sign of vulnerability or incompetence. It is common for women to resist showing vulnerability and asking for help, which can leave them dealing with daily stresses and challenges alone. Despite facing limitations and obstacles, many women are inclined to help others but resist asking for help for themselves. It has become a habit to take care of others, and neglect taking care of themselves. However, this behavior of taking care of others may not necessarily stem from feeling a sense of love, but rather from societal expectations and ingrained habits. Despite their unwavering strength, many Black women may experience overwhelming feelings of guilt and worthlessness when they sacrifice too much of themselves or fail to meet unrealistic expectations placed upon them. As a result, they may feel incomplete and unfulfilled.

When I met Yadira, she felt she was in a good place in her life. She had just bought a townhouse in the city and felt good about it. As I walked up the steps to her door, I saw a planter with a beautiful plant on the porch and a wreath on the door. She greeted me warmly when I rang her doorbell, and I entered a very pleasant and well decorated home. Her sixteen-year-old son came through and was very polite as he spoke to me before leaving to go and visit a friend. We sat at her kitchen table, and she told me about her life.

She shared that there was a time when she didn't feel good about herself, and she did not like her facial features or her body.

Two years prior to our meeting, she divorced her husband of seven years. He was seeing other women, which caused her to have negative thoughts about herself. She explained that she felt it was God who opened her eyes to her husband's inappropriate behavior. She started praying and working in the church, which helped her to love who she is and to become confidant in herself.

Yadira also stated that she felt a sense of confidence as she considered the effect of religion in her life:

> It [religion] makes me feel confident and the person or the woman that God has created me to be. We are all different. We all come to the table with different qualities and different skill sets and different backgrounds and different knowledge, so my faith in God and my belief in God at this point allow me to be confident in the woman that I have become and the woman that God has created me to be.

Several of the women acknowledged that religion enabled them to grasp and discover a new sense of personal dignity and meaning in their lives. Ada shared what religion had done for her:

> It [religion] makes me feel excellent about me. I am a black African queen. I am beautiful. I mean I look at the mirror and tell myself I feel sexy. I am sexy. I am me. I am who I am. . . . I just want to be myself and not nobody else or imitate nobody or look like nobody. I want to look like me for the person that I am. With God in my life today I feel good about myself as a person, as a woman.

Ada is forty-nine years old and has a long history of trauma. She lives in subsidized housing and supports herself through disability income. Her apartment is very small. She gave me a stool and I sat in the kitchen where she stood during the interview. She is a thin woman with a big smile and was very anxious to talk to me about her life. She reported that both her mother and grandmother are HIV positive. She has a history of drug addiction and stated that she no longer did drugs but did drink every now and then. She reported that she went into a faith-based drug addiction program that had a profound impact on her life. She felt empowered as she studied the Bible through the program, which enabled her know herself better and thus feel better about herself. She talked about how children so often come to her apartment and she feeds them. She feels strengthened as she acknowledges that God uses her to be a healer.

Rachel responded that her life had changed, and she felt "the best" since she had begun integrating religion into her life. When Rachel was younger, she did not feel good about herself due to her appearance. She acquired a new sense of value regarding herself since she had engaged with religion.

> [I feel] the best. At one point too and I would think too when I was younger when my mom and my dad divorced, even when I was young too because I was thinking it's like the society they put like a stipulation on certain people, like if you're dark skinned or you've got nappy hair or dah, dah, dah, so I didn't feel good about myself. But once I accepted Jesus Christ it's like there is nobody better than me, light skinned, dark skinned, long hair, short hair whatever, nobody. I don't care how much money you have, where you live at, whatever, no one is better than me.

Kelly described how when she was in college, she felt very isolated, her religion was not real for her, and she did not feel good about herself. In sharing her story, she spoke of a major transition when she felt suicidal and felt she got a sign from God that indicated how important she was:

> I knew that that day when my, well, fast-forward from that into the period of me wanting to take my life and having my friends come and knock on the door, it's like God is listening and it's at that point that it stopped being a religion that was my parents' religion, and it became personal for me, like you really understand me, me and God . . . I guess like when a person is able to really understand the fact that God loves them, like that mental well-being, it's something mentally, where you feel like you're not alone, well for me. When I got that part, it's like a light bulb just went off in my head, because it's like one thing to hear it and to be preached, hear sermons on top of sermons, but it's like when it really connects like, Kelly you're important. Like you have something to offer, you have something to give, and it's at that point that I believed that.

Paying attention to the stories of these women can give one

insight into what religion can do for an individual. For example, religion can be the groundwork that provides a sense of purpose for an individual by providing guidance on how to have a meaningful and fulfilling life. This sense of purpose for many has resulted in their serving others. In addition, some take on an intentional responsibility to improve themselves through prayer and meditation. Religion also can provide values and principles with which the individual can evaluate themselves, and then be guided by them in making decisions and actions. Religion also makes women feel good about themselves, which gives them new motivation to move forward in their lives without fear.

For many women, religion can transform their self-identity. Their beliefs and practices may become a central part of their lives, which will shape their worldview, values, and attitudes towards themselves and others. For those who connect with a church, temple or mosque, religion can provide a sense of community with shared identity and purpose. This can become deeply meaningful and fulfilling in individual's lives. Religion can influence not only their decision making, but also their behavior and their relationships with others, thus further contributing to their overall self-identity, one that encompasses and experiences empowerment.

Eight

The Mirror of the Media

While religion has historically been a positive resource for Black women in their day to day lives, the impact of historical trauma of the American slave system on generations of African Americans cannot be ignored. Gendered racism of Black women comes out of the history of white supremacy and patriarchy in this country. Stereotypes of Black women that have endured for centuries are those of the Jezebel, Mammy, Sapphire, and even the Black Super Woman. These images of Black women have followed them from slavery and continue to perpetuate themselves within religion, public policy, and public opinion and in the media.

During the era of slavery, a derogatory stereotype known as Jezebel or the "bad-black girl" emerged from the oppressive conditions in which white slave owners held absolute authority over the sexual agency and reproductive autonomy of Black women. The Jezebel image depicts the Black woman as a malevolent temptress known for her unconstrained promiscuous sexuality. This racist image portrayed the woman with more European features, often of mixed race, and with curly or straight hair. Black women were often subjected to societal pressures that emphasized conformity to the white standard of beauty, particularly during the time of slavery when white slave owners wielded significant influence over their lives and bodies. She is seen as over-sexed, and her only power is in her body and the influence she has over men.

The Mammy image was most famously portrayed by Hattie McDaniel in the film Gone With The Wind, though it repeatedly featured in other films. The Mammy stereotype is generally portrayed as a darker skinned, heavy woman, often a maid focused on taking care of everyone, especially her assigned white family. She works long, self-sacrificing hours, is asexual, and conforms to the expectations of her continued role as caregiver. She is only present to support the family she serves and has no real life of her own.

Another stereotype is the Sapphire, which is widely portrayed in television. The Sapphire is outspoken and quick-witted, often engaging in verbal exchanges that can undermine the confidence or authority of her husband, which perpetuates stereotypes about Black women emasculating men. She shows up as the angry Black woman who is sassy and doesn't take anything from anyone. The name derives from the character Sapphire, the wife of Kingfish in the Amos 'n' Andy television show.

These stereotypes continue to show up in print, film, internet, and social media. A response to these negative racist caricatures of Black women has been that of the Black Superwoman. The Superwoman image was developed to emphasize the often disregarded virtues, abilities, talents, and strengths that African American women possess in the face of oppression and hardship. The social and political lives of African American women are affected by gender-based discrimination, racism, marginalization, and inadequate resources. During and after slavery, these women were required to undertake the roles of mother, nurturer, and breadwinner. Becoming a Superwoman was critical for survival. Factors that also influenced this role were the marginalized and demeaned station of African American men, which limited their capacity to fulfil their families' needs.

African American women have often been commended for their strength and resilience. This has sometimes turned out to be a double-edged sword. On the one hand, these women have contributed to the health and growth of the African American community over many years. However, exerting too much effort and strength can result in stress and burnout. It is problematic that women find themselves working so hard for their families and communities that they forget about themselves. Another factor in Womanism is that it is spiritualized. Getting in touch with the Spirit that sustains them has often been an empowering tool in the use of prayer, worship and reading spiritual material including the bible and other spiritual texts. However, women must be careful that they do not find themselves working so hard for their families and in the community, and then find themselves also over-worked in the faith community. What these women do in working so hard for God in all the spheres of their lives can also lead to more stress and break down of health which can lead to depression, anxiety, and other mental health disorders.

The women in my study were looking at what contributed to their mental well-being. For many, balance in life was important to them to maintain a sense of peace and get rid of stress. Some thought that the remedy lie in changing their mindset, their attitude, and their perspective about life. Others were more focused on directly attending to their mental health by receiving mental health services. So much of their positive mental well-being had to do with how they tried to take care of themselves. Many Black women look to social media to learn the various ways to care for self with the newest information.

Social media for Black women has had a constructive impact. Black American women are among the largest consumer groups of social media in the United States. Recently Black women have populated social media platforms to exchange ideas about what it means to be a Black woman, and to resist systemic racism and gender oppression. Black women also use social media as an outlet for entertainment and information. With this interest in social media, it can therefore hold significant emotional meaning for women and become deeply integrated into their lives. This does not come without risk, however. It is very possible that one can become addicted to this outlet.

The impact of mainstream beauty standards has negatively affected Black women, whether it is portrayed on television or social media. Black women's features are customarily rejected by the mainstream and seen as masculine and undesirable. European attributes have been seen as America's standard of beauty. Within Black families and the African American community, lighter complected persons often have more advantages and obtain higher education and career success. As noted, mainstream American culture prizes straight or loose curls, while historically traditional Black hairstyles have resulted in people losing their jobs or place at school. In an Instagram survey, 134 Black women were surveyed with the majority believing that they have been discriminated against because of their skin color, texture of their hair, or African features. The #BlackGirlMagic social media movement has done much to impact the self-esteem of Black girls and women. Within this movement, Black women are embracing their natural hair and the beauty of their darker skin color and African features.

Broadcast religious media has a long history in the African American community on both television and radio. Research has shown that African Americans watch religious television programs at a greater rate than non-Hispanic whites. There has been much speculation regarding the high involvement of African Americans in both religious organization and religious print and media. In looking at the plight of Black people in this country, with racism and white supremacy rearing their ugly heads again in new ways, it is understandable that just as so many looked to religion and spirituality during the civil rights era this practice continues today.

In 2014, television news stations showed activists challenging church leaders after the killing of Michael Brown. What became the Black Lives Matter movement criticized the church with its homophobia, misogyny, and hypocrisy. Internet articles addressed young people's concerns about religious leaders apparent apathy. They felt the church had failed to address systemic racism. Racism and white supremacy still have a hold on white Christianity in this country. Young people all over the country became activists, which for some represented a form of active spirituality. The press, social media, television news, and internet articles shed light on the matter of the church not being involved in addressing shootings of young Black men.

White Evangelical Christianity has taken a hold on this nation with its conservative views and fundamentalist reading of the biblical text. The news media's conservative stations, such as Fox News, have contributed to this narrative, which has led to a stacked conservative Supreme Court taking away women's rights to control their own bodies. Black and Brown women are most affected by abortion bans, as they are often not able to travel out of state to address these health needs. In addition, the mandated and approved programs granting special consideration to historically excluded groups, specifically racial minorities, or women, have now been wiped out by the Supreme Court. These programs focused on access to education and employment, and the change continues to reek of racism for the Black community.

Sometimes the media can be used to promote positive messaging. In 2007 my husband and I conducted Holy Union services for a gay couple and a lesbian couple. Afterwards, a Washington Post reporter interviewed congregation members and wrote a large article that appeared on the front page of the newspaper's metro section entitled "Rift Over Gay Unions Reflects New Battle to Black Churches." The article addressed our theological stance and engaged with the congregation members' statements. It also addressed how many Black churches see homosexuality as a sin and forbid any religious rituals for same-sex couples. In response, many community newspaper articles and social media posts condemned our inclusivity. On the other hand, some progressive white churches and Open and Affirming churches reached out to us. We were aware of the discrimination and hurt, emotionally and spiritually, of our Black gay and lesbian brothers and sisters. I sat in my office counseling many of these persons who were harmed by the attitude of the church. They often shed tears over feeling worthless, and some were on the brink of suicide. I was able to refer several women and men to therapists who were affirming of the LGBTQ community because so many have struggled with poor mental health due to abuse and discrimination from the church. In another article that my husband the Rev Dr. Dennis Wiley and I wrote for the Washington Post in the same year, we stated that "we as African Americans, should be the last people in the world based on our history, to turn around and oppress others."

In another Washington Post article written in 2021 with the title "The Black Church Must Reckon with How It Has Treated Its Queer Members," Ashton Crawley states that queerness in the Black community and in the church has always existed and the question now is how can the church move forward with honesty and love. The church has the chance to move forward and show people how to be together in difference.

Some progressive Christian denominations do affirm the LGBTQ community, such as The United Church of Christ, Disciples of Christ, The Alliance of Baptists, More Light Presbyterians, Reconciling Ministries of the United Methodist Church, Metropolitan Community Churches, The Episcopal Church, The Convergent Catholic Communion and other groups and denominations have done much to address anti-racism and also affirm LGBTQ+ individuals. The numbers of African Americans in these groups, however, are scant compared to those in traditional Black churches. Their social media and newsletters provide educational and affirming information regarding the LGBTQ community. In contrast, the major Black Church denominations have held on tightly to homophobia and heterosexism with small change over the years, which traumatizes and hurts gay individuals psychologically and spiritually. Denominations such as African Methodist Episcopal (AME) African Methodist Episcopal Zion (AMEZ), Christian Methodist Episcopal (CME), Church of God in Christ (COGIC) National Baptist Convention of America Inc. (NBCA), National Baptist Convention U.S.A., Inc. (NBC), National Missionary Baptist Convention of America (NMBCA), and Progressive National Baptist Convention (PNBC) have churches who bash LGBTQ people in the pulpit, do not mention this group at all, or preach that all need Jesus but need to give up their sinful behavior. Those churches who are more open to the gay, lesbian, and trans community may often preach and teach an inclusive gospel but fall short of making this a church policy of becoming open and affirming of the LGBTQ community.

The way the Black church generally treats LGBTQ persons does lead to stress, anxiety, depression and other mental health symptoms for these individuals if they are trying to become a part of these fellowships. "Coming out" as a Black person takes much courage and risk. A movement that has alleviated stress of these individuals has been Black church denominations and congregations that are open and affirming and largely headed by gay pastors and bishops such as The Fellowship of Affirming Ministries (TFAM), and Unity Fellowship Church Movement (UFCM). Whether it is overt racism, or internalized oppression by Black people themselves, these can bring on both physical and mental health concerns. More needs to happen in print media, film, social media, podcasts, and other venues to lift up positivity and inclusion of this community. However, even as both Black women and the LGBTQ community have faced discrimination in our society, and as much as things remain the same, they also change. There is positive movement in that Black women and Black same gender loving people serve as journalists both in print, television, podcasts and other venues. However, at the same time there are positive offerings in the media, very conservative journalism continues to denigrate these individuals.

Nine

The Spiritual Journeys of Black Men

Black men have diverse experiences of and perspectives on religion and spirituality. For some Black men, Christianity is a central aspect of their religious and spiritual lives. However, there is a wide range of spiritual beliefs within the Black community including various forms of Islam, Judaism, African traditional religions, and other faiths. These diverse religious practices reflect the rich cultural heritage and global connections of Black communities. In addition, spirituality can also be expressed outside of organized religion. Some Black men may engage in practices such as meditation, mindfulness, yoga, or ancestral reverence to connect with their inner selves and find meaning in their lives.

The experiences of Black men with religion and spirituality are affected by age, geographic location, socioeconomic status, and personal experience. All these factors shape the individual's beliefs and practices. How does Black men's spirituality connect with that of Black women? Some Black women who I have worked with expressed frustration at the reluctance of their husbands or men in their families to take on the role of spiritual leader. This may come from cultural or societal expectations and gender roles that place the importance of strong male leadership in the family. Some Black women feel that their partners or males within the family are not involved in their own spiritual development, or are just refusing to become the spiritual head because it is uncomfortable. Personal beliefs of men, as well as their upbringing and experiences, can factor into whether they are willing to take on these roles. The notion that men are not "leading their families spiritually" could contribute to the false generalization that Black men are ambivalent towards religion and spirituality.

What often is not addressed is the number of Black men who are deeply spiritual and involved in religion. According to the Pew Research Center, men in general are as a rule less religious than women. However, a significant number of Black men maintain strong religious beliefs. As a matter of fact, Black men are more religious than white men, white women, and Hispanic men, and have the same rates of religiosity as Hispanic women. However, some scholars have observed that Black men are not as religiously involved as Black women. Research indicates that low levels of religious involvement for men increased the probability of depressive symptoms.

It has been a scientific puzzle as to why women are generally more religious in this country than men, but there are various theories. One posits that testosterone makes men more willing to take more risks and gamble that they will not face punishment in an afterlife, and that they are less religious for this reason, while women are more risk-averse and lean to religion to assure a place in heaven. Other researchers feel that some genetic factors that are tied to unknown psychological aspects may account for the variation between men and women, such as physical, or physiological causes such as genes, hormones or biological predispositions. In contrast, some researchers assert that socialization into the conventional gender roles, economic structures in the United States, and somewhat lower rates of women in the workforce account for the difference. Conclusive evidence that would settle this nature versus nurture dispute over the differences in religiosity between men and women seems to be lacking, however. Even though there has been much cultural and societal change, the gender gap in religion still endures. It appears that perhaps the differences arise from the convoluted mix of many causes at the same time.

When it comes to specifically looking at the differences in Black men and women, Black women have greater rates of participation in both organized and non-organized religious life. One example is prayer. The National Survey of Black Americans indicates that 68% of Black men pray every day, whereas 84% of Black women pray every day.

As we look at the reasons for these differences between Black men and women, the social and family arena points to women as those who are the caregivers with a nurturing role. They are the principal individuals who socialize children and share teaching around ethical behavior and religious values. In addition, the multiple roles that women have such as wife, mother, worker, and caregiver, increase their stress levels and often they must employ religious coping skills to make it from day to day.

For Black people, this nation has been one of trauma, heartache, poverty, and turmoil amid chattel slavery, segregation, discrimination, racism, white supremacy, and poverty. The memories of the abduction, torture, and lynching of Emmett Till in the Jim Crow South are still in the threads of our nation as we also remember George Floyd, another Black man among others who was murdered by white privilege, violence, and the police. Mass incarceration of Black men over the years has grown exponentially, with Black men disproportionally represented in the prison system. When we look at religion and Black men, we must also include those who are incarcerated. The Muslim religion, especially the Nation of Islam, has had a significant impact on incarcerated Black men. Some African Americans reacted to the images of a white Jesus and identified, instead, with the Honorable Elijah Muhammed who led the Nation of Islam from 1934 until his death in 1975. Although this faith was heavily tied to Black Nationalism, there was also a heavy emphasis on self-help, racial unity, and discipline among its members. While it is important to note that not all Black men in prison are Muslim, and certainly not all Black Muslims have been incarcerated, there is a significant presence of Black men who have embraced Islam while incarcerated.

In prison, religion can play a crucial role in providing solace, guidance, and a sense of community for individuals. For some Black men, the Nation of Islam offered a spiritual path that resonates with their life experiences and provides a framework for personal growth and transformation. Black men often identify with the teachings of Islam, such as discipline, self-reflection, and accountability. This can help individuals to navigate the challenges of prison life and help them to live their daily lives if they have been wrongly charged and incarcerated, or to grapple with any wrong they have done. Islam can also offer a sense of identity and belonging for many Black men in prison. It can provide a connection to their rich cultural heritage and provide a community that supports and understands their struggles. Empowerment, resilience, and a renewed sense of purpose can be found in the practice of Islam. Within this religion there has been an emphasis on social justice and equality that resonates with Black men who have experienced systemic racism and injustice. This emphasis can sometimes inspire them to advocate for change both within the prison system and society at large. Many men involved with The Nation of Islam engage in educational programs, mentorship, and community service to uplift themselves and others. I do recognize, however, that the experiences of Black men, prison, and Islam are not monolithic. Every person's journey is unique, shaped by personal circumstances, cultural backgrounds, and individual choices. Some Black men find solace in other religious or spiritual practices, while others may not engage in religion at all.

Because of racism in the society and violence toward Black people, especially Black men, historically men have often not received opportunities for upward mobility. Women have had to step up in the culture to work, take care of children, and often take on the role of religious and spiritual educator and leader. The Black Church is overwhelmingly made up of women, which also contributes to the stereotype of Black men having ambivalence regarding religion and spirituality. Some men who embrace the role of leader in the family sometimes erroneously misinterpret scripture and feel that they must make every decision and tell their partners what to do. This has often led to a man becoming a perpetrator of domestic violence. The Biblical admonition "wives obey your husbands" has often been misused and has contributed to the intimate partner violence along with misogyny towards women.

It is important to consider the historical and cultural factors that have shaped the dynamics that lead to Black women being frustrated that Black men will not be spiritual leaders in their families. This shift can be attributed to different influences such as increased access to information, changing gender roles, and the changing modern ideologies. As a result, some Black men may choose to explore alternative sources for understanding themselves, such as personal experiences, education, self-reflection, or seeking guidance from mentors and role models outside of religious or spiritual contexts.

It is important that Black families and Black communities understand cultural change and learn to recognize individual choice and autonomy. Fostering open and honest communication within families will allow for discussions about spirituality, values, and the roles that family members want to embrace. Hopefully, the result will be the creation of an environment where everyone feels supported and empowered to explore their own paths to self-understanding and fulfillment.

Ten

Nurturing Young Souls

What does it mean for Black mothers who tend to have the responsibility of leading, guiding and giving moral education to their children? Although there are many Black families with committed husbands and fathers, the vast majority (72%) of Black children are born to single mothers, a rate that surpasses the rates of all other ethnic groups in the United States. Dr. Natalie Carroll, an obstetrician in Houston, Texas, advocates for girls to get married citing that two parents are needed to give children what they need. Statistics show that children of unmarried mothers of any race are more likely to underperform in school, be poor as adults, do drugs, go to prison, and have their own children out of wedlock. In the Black community, I feel that single parenthood is not a deficiency but, instead, shows forth the resilience of women who learn to engage with a community of mothers because of an unavailability of suitable men as fathers, whether they are in prison or unequipped to be present as a father for various reasons.

Mothers who have a career also have the responsibility of moving between their job and their children's school and activities and home responsibilities. Many Black mothers—regardless of their socioeconomic status—experience guilt because they feel that they do not spend enough time with their children . In addition, mothers experience fears that their children will face police violence, White supremacy, racism, microaggressions, and the stresses placed on Black children by society. Added to these mothers' concerns for their children is that their own children may become teen mothers. Although the number of teen mothers is declining, for Black and Hispanic girls the rates are still much higher than for White girls. Confronting all of these issues, how do mothers ensure that their children are safe while providing them with guidance and nurturing them so that they can become whole individuals? Whole individuals become aware of their own spirituality and can discern whether there is a religious path they may want to follow that will help them.

Teen mothers need significant support to care for their babies. A study conducted by Brown, Caldwell and Antonucci explored the connection between conflict in Black and White mother-daughter relationships, the impact of attending religious services and activities, and depression. They noted that it is essential for a teenage mother to have the support of her mother, the baby's grandmother, so that the teenager will feel supported, feel good about herself, and feel she is effective in the care of her child. Sometimes, however, while the teenager is adjusting to motherhood, conflicts can arise between the new mom and the grandmother regarding parenting styles, and the values and goals of the teen's belief systems, including how she wants to raise her child.

But the study demonstrated that religious services and activities could help connect mothers and daughters. Attending a religious service where there are people with similar values, beliefs, customs, and hopes, appeared to positively affect relationships between mothers and teenage and reduce conflict. One reason revolves around the community support provided by participating in church or religious activities. Moreover, religious beliefs can serve as a coping mechanism which can lessen conflict, reduce stress, and prevent depression.

The researchers found that Black grandmothers had higher levels of belief than White grandmothers. However, Black grandmothers experienced more conflict with their daughters who were teenage mothers than White mothers did. The researchers felt that attending religious services and activities together could serve as a buffer in these relationships. Nevertheless, Black grandmothers with higher levels of religiosity also reported higher levels of depression than White grandmothers, which could influence their availability to support their daughters. Lower levels of depression in White grandmothers may have been a result of more sources of support and higher income, according to the researchers. Notwithstanding, higher levels of religious belief and attending religious activities for both White and Black grandmothers were associated with less depression. This again points to religion and its activities serving as coping mechanisms regardless of race.

While Patricia Hill Collins does not specifically speak to spirituality or religion, she addresses the fact that from slavery until modern times, oppressive conditions for Black women have not allowed them to fit into a Eurocentric model of motherhood. In her essay "The Meaning of Motherhood in Black Culture and Black Mother/Daughter Relationships," Collins asked her students, "What did your mother teach you about men?" Amongst various answers the students stressed their mothers' "insistence on being self-reliant and resourceful." Historically, Black women have had to work outside of the home in a limited number of occupations, which conflicted with caring for children. This led to the establishment of communities of mothers, who often saw themselves as responsible for one another's children. "Other mothers," whether relatives or not, often looked out for children, sometimes taking them in when their biological mothers were not available.

In the AARP report "Grandparents Raising Grandchildren in the District of Columbia: Focus Group Report," the authors noted that grandparents raising grandchildren is increasing nationwide. Black and Hispanic heads of households are considerably more likely to feel a sense of obligation to their grandchildren than Whites. There are some differences in the way grandparents have received their grandchildren. Some have felt forced into the role because of the death of their children or by the legal or welfare system. Many are stressed and angry due to the situation they find themselves in. Many have feelings of inadequacy, inability to receive adequate income (foster care providers receive substantially more than grandparents taking care of their grandchildren), along with an inadequate educational system and mental health services. In addition to anger, grandparents may experience guilt, depending on the circumstances. Many do portray their faith, family support, and the church as being helpful to them.

As I think about myself as a Black mother of now three grown children I reflect on my life and motherhood. When my children were young, I remember as a working mother feeling so guilty when I felt I was not spending enough time with them. Ten years separated my eldest daughter Aiyana and my next child Samira. My eldest was the product of my first marriage. I remarried when I was 35 and gave birth to Samira at the age of 37 and Joshua at the age of 39. I was ordained as a minister a year before Samira was born, and eventually left the position of Clinical Administrator in the Inpatient Child and Adolescent Psychiatric Services Division of a mental health hospital. I remember struggling because I was a new minister, a neophyte, and a woman on church staff, whereas before this I was a very seasoned and comfortable leader working in the field of mental health. I was also a wife, a mother, and a student in a Doctor of Ministry program in pastoral psychotherapy. At the same time, I was also having to wrestle with some of the demons and trauma of my childhood—sexual abuse by my stepfather.

Like so many Black mothers, I sought healing and guidance not only from a therapist, but also from my faith. I am one of the 75% of African Americans who identify as Christians and there is a reason for this. This is the faith I was introduced to as a young child, and the one in which I made a deep connection in my spirituality to God.

Going back to slavery Africans came from different tribes with different languages, different food, and different cultures. Many came as Muslims and with African Traditional Religions, but they were able to appropriate Christianity to fit who they were. Embracing their own version of Christianity was something that pulled them together. They took the religion of the oppressor and changed it, making it their own with their own music and culture. They saw the religion as liberating as they became aware of the Israelites being held in slavery, and God leading them out of bondage. They identified with this story for it gave them hope. African culture remains a part of Black Christianity as worshipers in church can "feel the religion" and there is an emotional response. For Black people in many places of worship it is an "embodied" religion. This means there may be expressive praise and music, the "shout," call and response, and in many cases dancing in the spirit.

It is true that when some young people graduate from high school and/or college they may neglect attending church only to return later when they have children. That certainly is the case with me as I became active in the church again when my first child was 18 months old. As I noted previously, I had a relationship with God, with the Spirit, and had a spiritual life. When I had my first daughter, I thought about how necessary it was going to be for her to have a felt connection with her own spirituality and her own relationship. She, as well as I, needed a way to trust our own intuition. So often Black women are growing and recovering from their own internal trauma as they raise their children and try to teach them to reach without and within to a higher power.

Black mothers love their children and for generations have sensed a need to bring the ethics of spirituality to them. Today many young Black mothers struggle to find a place where they and their children fit in. Many mothers are attracted to the notion of mindfulness meditation with its benefits for the body, the mind, and the spirit. However, for their young children, mothers are wanting a sense of community where children enjoy and can participate in the songs and music, prayers, and rituals. The truth is that now many mothers are seeking a more contemplative kind of religion that teaches principles and precepts, but at the same time, they love the history and experience of the Black Church minus the exclusion and judgment of the church. In her book, We Live for the We: The Political Power of Black Motherhood, Dani McClain, a Black mother, says, "I believe that Buddhism offers the clearest, most compelling teachings on the nature of the mind and that Christianity—as analyzed by the likes of Howard Thurman and Thomas Merton—offers the clearest, most compelling teachings on love." Kim Tabari shares about teaching her young son about meditation by finding child focused instruction on-line. She sits with him and starts with just five minutes and increases it from time to time in two-minute intervals. She teaches her son that even a small amount of daily meditation will improve his health. She tells her son it can be helpful for him to figure out why he feels like he feels.

Black mothers play a significant role in the development of their children's spiritual and religious life. In many parts of the Black community, spirituality and religion have been fundamental ingredients of this community and are seen as valuable and essential in raising well developed children. These mothers see it as their responsibility to pass on their religious background and practices to their children to develop a positive foundation for their spiritual growth.

For many Black mothers, spirituality and religion provide a sense of identity for their children which grounds them and provides them with strength and resilience. The insidious attacks that children face today, from microaggressions in the community at large to gun violence by police and racist messaging on social media, can negatively impact them if they are not given something that can aid them from within. Black mothers can instill in their children a deep belief in God which allows the children to draw on their faith during times of adversity. Children learn to draw on their religious teaching and spirituality to traverse the trials and injustices that they may experience.

Just as in any culture, there is diversity in the Black community. Not all Black mothers and children practice religion in the same manner. There are some who practice faiths other than Christianity in the Black Church tradition, such as Islam, those who adhere to Black Nationalism and African Traditional Religious practice, East Asian religious practices, as well as those who have a more individualistic and personal approach to spirituality. It is clear, however, that Black mothers play a central role in the cultivation of their children's religious and spiritual development, which helps the children to discern their own values and beliefs.

It is also noteworthy to understand that not all religious instruction has been a good model for Black children. Black children have been adversely impacted by the foundations of a religious identity in several ways. Stereotypes and prejudices within the teaching of scriptural texts due to misinterpretation such as representing Black people as innately inferior or sinful can lead to shame and low self-esteem in Black children. In addition, the religious traditions that adhere to strict gender roles or say that the LGBTQ community is sinful can be extremely damaging to those children who do not fit into these norms. These practices can cause estrangement from the religious community.

It is the calling of mothers to instill in their children a deeper sense of who they are as individuals, and how God created them and loves them just as they are. Sharing positive stories and messages to remind children of their worth and value and to embrace their uniqueness and diversity is important. Mothers can teach children to stand up for themselves in the face of injustice and encourage self-empathy for their children and for others, including understanding and respect for everyone. Mothers who show demonstrative love and care for their children help the children to love themselves, to love others, and to love God.

Eleven

Making a Way Out of No Way

What gets old but never ages? The stories of Black women. Their prayers, doubts, suffering, resilience, and joys have never aged since the time they were brought against their will to this country, a place of unseen dangers and tragedy. Survival has been a theme that Black women have carried, often forgetting about themselves. Bearing the responsibility of surviving for others, their children and family members, and their community, they have hoped that those they lived for might do more than survive but might even thrive.

In the Black community there are different stories and different levels of experience and trauma, but the same sense of pain and sacrifice that Black women have had to endure. So often, only calling on the name of Jesus that has been able to bring some sense of relief. Women have found themselves in systems where justice has been denied. Often their only recompense has been to call on God. In that calling, something can happen within them, a connection with the Spirit that bolsters them and empowers them to keep on keeping on, making a way out of no way. This becomes a coping mechanism for them, one that generations of Black women have used, calling on the Spirit to assist them and hold them when there is no imminent change in their lives.

In addressing spirituality, some have seen a difference in how white women and Black women interpret their experience with Jesus. In her 1989 book, White Women's Christ and Black Women's Jesus: Feminist Christology and Womanist Response, Jacquelyn Grant states that feminist writers of Christology (a branch of theology that addresses the nature and work of Jesus Christ) have only considered the experiences of white women and not women of color or non-western women. In the same vein, Black theology did not address the perspective of Black women. Grant's response is that of womanist theology that comes out of Black women's experience and explores the truth of present-day Black women.

African slaves also gave their own perspective of the person of Jesus. They reinterpreted Christianity for themselves and were strengthened by the determination and endurance of Jesus as he went through torture. They found hope in his resurrection and this hope continues today in the Black community's ongoing struggle for equality amid racism and white supremacy. As we look at the culture in our country today, it appears as if we are going backwards and haywire at the same time. White supremacy continues to rear its ugly head, evangelical Christians are supporting a very conservative ideology and ignoring the least, the lost, and the left out. Diversity, Equity, and Inclusion programs are being shut down all over the country because of legislation passed by the Republican Party. Roe v. Wade was overturned by the Supreme Court, and Affirmative Action programs in colleges and universities are gone.

Even as Black people and Black women pray to be protected from unseen dangers, it seems as if justice is hiding. There has been a slight decline in the poverty rate for Black individuals, but racial inequities still exist (census.gov). The stresses of everyday life added to the inequalities of American culture are what must be negotiated and dealt with in a manner that results in people being well and whole.

The quest for being well and whole is what the women in this study were seeking. For many of the women in this study, it became apparent that their mental well-being did not mean that they were without stress. The stressors did not define them, but forced them to use coping skills, many of which came from their religious toolbox. I was amazed at Mary Beth and her story. She was told that she would die at the age of 18 and had been living with AIDS and other illnesses for 25 years at the time of the interview. She was living in poverty and wanted to move but it was not yet happening for her. When I asked her how religion made her feel about her life and how it has affected her, she said it made her feel great because she knew God loved her more than her mother loved her, and for her it was a wonderful feeling. "It makes you feel like you are special, like you are one of a kind." She used meditation and prayer, which helped her in her day-to-day life.

Like Mary Beth, Becky also attended a clinic and felt that her mental well-being had much to do with seeing a therapist and being involved in the church as a minister. She too had experienced trauma in her life and was a survivor of domestic violence. She also felt that God had healed her from her medical and mental health issues.

Rachel was a very busy pastor and felt that her religion connected with her mental well-being by keeping her grounded. She felt her study and reading kept her balanced even when there were very difficult times in her life. Balance was a theme for her and several of the women who felt that balance was necessary for good mental well-being, and they could get this when engaged in prayer, or reading spiritual material, meditation, or worship. I know myself when I settle down to journal or read scripture or have a devotional time, I also feel a sense of calm, and I can often give my concerns to God. It does not mean that I will be absent of stress, but that I can still go forward with hope amid difficulty that my issue will be resolved, or if not, God's presence will allow me to stay grounded and well. Often Black preachers will quote Psalm 30:5, "Weeping may endure for a night, but joy comes in the morning" (NKJV). We must be careful, for the night of slavery lasted for over 400 years, and oppression and injustice continue to this day.

Another woman in the study, Eartha, was clearly impacted by the systemic oppression of her impoverished community. She was very clear that her hope came from attending church. She was an alcoholic and a widow with five children. She felt that it was not the social worker or the psychologist but the church and its members that ministered to her and loved her and helped her get sober. Her church was very involved in recovery ministry. She felt that the church pointed her to God. She said, "It was a process, religion made me learn and taught me that I'm a child of God, of the most high and that He has things for me to do."

Tynisha's experience was different. She was disappointed with "organized religion." Tynisha, a 50-year-old social worker, shared that religion for her was the practice of Buddhism which gave her peace. She also attended group therapy to help her deal with the stresses of her everyday life. She talked about reading a range of religious materials and listening to television pastors. She says she does not go to church because she knows the history of Christianity, which is disturbing, and she feels there is a lot of corruption in the church. I have found that many who do not profess a religion or belong to a faith community within the Black community will still tell you that they believe in God and that they pray.

Linda, a 43-year-old social worker, is also ambivalent about organized religion. She believes in counseling and therapy but feels many of the people she knows rely on their faith only and she feels that they may also need mental health care. She revealed that she suffers from depression and has sought mental health care. She says she goes to church every now and then but doesn't really feel comfortable and wonders if there is really a God. Yet, something still draws her to wonder and sometimes pray.

Yadira, who also recalls having been depressed, feels that the church just says you must have faith. Only recently has she experienced in her current church education and a positive attitude towards mental health care, which she finds encouraging. She does have some uncertainty, however, about both being in therapy and the church. She has positive thoughts and feelings about both, but she is also in a quandary when discussing religion and mental well-being. What is interesting is that she is an ordained minister in her church.

Black women are not monolithic in their discernment of faith. As the title of this book suggests, "Don't JUST give me that old time religion." One size does not fit all. Acknowledging that Black women are the most religious people in this country means also acknowledging that their interpretations of religion may differ from one another. Women were typically the ones who ensured that societal customs and practices were preserved in the church. However, patriarchy needs both men and women to keep it going. Some women felt uneasy about the roles women were assigned in the church, which allowed them to serve only in particular areas with deference to men. Some experienced a liberating God who met them where they were and did not judge them but empowered them. This empowerment allowed them to discern how they would practice religion, whether in the community of faith or out of it. Using coping skills, they learned to wait on God, and some left the church. In her book In My Grandmother's House: Black Women, Faith and the Stories We Inherit, Dr. Yolanda Pierce acknowledges that when there is no sense of love present in a family, a faith community or in a sermon "people will walk away."

Black women need to embrace themselves and seek places and resources that bring them wholeness. Some women did this by adding experiences such as meditation along with their participation in a faith community. Some were ambivalent and unsure whether it was better to stay or leave their faith community. Womanist theology is concerned with uplifting the community no matter who helps. Those churches that are only interested in individual religious devotion and practice can become devoid of meaning for the women who see Jesus as liberator of the least, the lost, and the left out. It is in these spaces that sometimes our physical presence can be there, but our minds are elsewhere.

It is true that church attendance and Christianity in this country are declining among all ethnicities and faith communities. Those who profess no faith or religion are on the rise. What we know, however, is that African Americans endured centuries of slavery by holding onto hope for a life that will help them to thrive and be whole in the face of struggle. In looking at the biblical text, it has been apparent that the ministry of Jesus has been on the side of the oppressed. Many of the women in this study have learned to affirm themselves, take gentle care of themselves, and love themselves in spite of all that they endure. Black women face obstacles due to their gender and their race whether educated or not, having a sustainable economic situation or not. As we look at the diaspora of Black people in this world, it is true that Black women are often in lower-paying positions, face higher poverty rates, and are consistently at a disadvantage when compared to white women. Black people have health disparities and are at higher risk of heart disease, stroke, cancer, asthma influenza, pneumonia, diabetes, HIV/AIDS, and COVID. Black women have the highest infant mortality rate of any group in this country. Irrespective of pain and difficulty in their lives, many Black women continue to have a hope and a faith that allows them to keep on going. Hebrews 11 contains a long list of those who did amazing things by using their faith. Yet it also says that so many were persecuted and tortured and discriminated against and killed just as so many in the Black community are persecuted and killed both within the community, and by police. Hebrews 11:39 states, "Yet all these, though they were commended for their faith, did not receive what was promised" (RSV). The promise for Black women is living a whole and healthy and good life. My hope and prayer is that in spite of injustice, even though those that belong to religious institutions is on the decline, that Black women will continue to lift themselves and their communities up, practicing their sense of what religion and spirituality means to them, and keep "making a way out of no way."

Twelve

Final Note for Helping Professionals

I am very grateful to the twenty women who gave their time to help me in this research. They did not know me in the beginning and took a risk to share with a stranger how they experienced religion in their lives. The findings of my study illustrate how these Black women understand the meaning of mental well-being and how their mental well-being connects with their perception of religion. Their understanding of mental well-being has much to do with their own personal history and experience. Their exposure to and familiarity with various aspects of their lives tends to influence how they define mental well-being. All the women in this study presented with their own challenges and experiences of stress. These women's sense of mental well-being has nothing to do with the absence of stress. They have learned how to manage their stress, especially with their use of religion. Their mental well-being is not the absence of stress at all, but the management of stress. Mental well-being for these women is dynamic, changing, and suited to wherever they are in their lives.

The twenty women who participated in this research provided insight and understanding into a subject matter that is often stereotyped and misunderstood. As a group in this country, Black women are understood as a marginalized group from a marginalized community. Although various studies have continued to show that Black women are the most religious group within the United States, this study does not support that all Black women are involved in traditional religion. The subjects of the study have different definitions for religion and what it means for them. Their involvement in religion varies in the intensity and the modality. One finding that needs more study is the interest in meditation. Studies have shown the efficacy of meditation for health and wellness, and it is apparent that some women, while being involved in traditional religion, are also engaged in meditation, even though their tradition may frown on it.

There appear to be no trends based on education, age, or socioeconomics or marital status. There are more commonalities than differences among the women. Income levels and education of these Black women may be higher than the general population due to their location in Washington, DC. However, research has shown that income above $75,000 per year does not necessarily increase well-being. There may be a general belief that increased income and education, marriage, and youth might improve overall mental well-being. The study did not demonstrate this. It is important to understand that the deep meaning religion holds for Black women has more bearing on mental well-being than these other factors. For these women, the experience of their religious faith emerges out of their struggle. From this struggle women can reflect and examine the various ways they are oppressed in multiple aspects of their lives. The women are often able to see God not only as a liberator, but as sustainer. They embrace a theology of survival. "God can make a way out of no way." This information may be helpful to recognize, especially if those working with Black women such as social workers and health providers can then design interventions to increase the mental well-being of Black women. Bringing the voices of Black women's definitions of both mental well-being and religion for them is important. It is important to note not only that religion is important for Black women, but also what religion is for Black women, and how is it helpful or not helpful.

Womanist theology and empowerment theory are the frameworks I used to understand Black women's experience and resilience in the face of challenges. While the findings of this study are not voluminous, they offer groundwork to further explore and study how Black women are able to find themselves empowered in the midst of difficulty, and how social workers, mental health providers, clergy and health providers can more effectively aid in this empowerment.

What I have learned based on the information gathered in this study is:

* Despite a decline in religion, religion is helpful and empowering for Black women.
* Mental well-being for Black women is not the absence of stress at all, but the management of stress.
* There is diversity in religious beliefs and practices among Black women; traditional religion is not necessarily the norm.
* Black women's understanding of mental well-being has much to do with their own personal history and experience.
* There are no trends based on education, age, socioeconomics, or marital status; however, there are more commonalities than differences among the women.

My journey through this research has been one of affirmation and empowerment. Even as religion and spirituality has been so significant for me in my life, I have had some discomfort in my own pilgrimage in the Black church, even as some of the women in this study were not completely comfortable in the Black Church. To hear their stories affirmed my own experience. The way many Black churches exclude and even demonize the LGBTQ community has stunned me. The thirty-two years that my husband and I pastored together has been one of openness and inclusion of all people. In the last thirteen years of our pastorate before retirement, our church became open and affirming of LGBTQ+ people, and in fact we performed our first Holy Union service in 2007 when at that time Massachusetts was the only state that had marriage equality. Two years later in 2009, we led 150 clergy in Washington, DC to sign a document affirming marriage equality which the city council stated helped them to change the DC laws to affirm marriage equality in 2010. The gay community including gay women are marginalized and often hurt by religion. As Linda, one of the women in the study, stated, she wasn't getting the answers and church was not giving her the meaning that she needed. Some parts of the church still do not allow women in some leadership positions such as deacons and clergy; this continues to marginalize women in the church.

The women in this study confirmed some of my uneasiness about Black church culture, but at the same time, they helped me understand that it was a place where I was able to grow spiritually. I resonate with some of the women as I explore other faith traditions such as Buddhism, and different worship styles and spiritualities. Even though I am a Christian and secure in my faith, I see other religions as a way human beings express their faith and devotion to a higher power. As I became acquainted with the diversity of how these women felt that religion impacted them, whether it had to do with experiencing the spirit in nature, in the church, in prayer, or meditation, it helped me not to put my religion or my experience of God in a box. Seeing the struggles of these women and how they used their religion and spirituality to cope in a positive manner was very freeing for me. I could also identify with those that were ambivalent, because I have been where they are. As a young woman, I remember asking "Is God really real?" My hope is that where they are is part of their process of deepening their own spirituality. As a social worker and clergy member, it is important for me to know how to introduce the concept of religion and spirituality to my clients using cultural competence. My inquiry will let me know if this is something that a client wants to incorporate in the work we do together.

Many social workers and clinicians involved in clinical practice are aware of the significance of religion and spirituality. In 2011, the Council on Social Work Education developed a committee called the CSWE Religion and Spirituality Work Group. Prior to this, CSWE curriculum policy statements identified religion as an area of diversity for study in social work education. The committee determined that knowing the culture and obtaining knowledge about a client's religion, in addition to possessing the skills to address it, is essential for social work practice.

Teaching about diverse spiritual traditions and interventions is clearly needed in the social work curriculum. The Educational Policy and Accreditation Standards (EPAS) (2015) of the Council on Social Work Education's (CSWE) second competency is to engage diversity and difference in practice. The many dimensions of diversity include but are not limited to age, color, class, ethnicity, race, and religion. Understanding the complexities of the many facets of diversity is important for social workers as they also manage their own prejudices and preconceptions. Understanding Black women, their conceptions of religion, and how they intersect with their mental well-being is central for social workers who work with this population.

Religion is a universal construct. Each religious tradition has its own sense of what religion and spirituality are and how they are manifested. It has its own traditions, diverse spiritualties, and the ethos of individual's lives. Social workers must work with cultural competency and comprehend how necessary it is to get the whole picture of an individual to understand the "person in environment," so that effective care can be given. The opportunity for the fulfillment of basic needs, well-being, and justice is necessary for all. It is commonly recognized that the culture has an obligation to provide information, education, and support to those who are marginalized. The same holds true for Black women. Black women can also feel the same poor mental health that is experienced by those who are disenfranchised. Cultural competency regarding the primacy of religion in the lives of Black women will help to develop the most effective interventions to aid in the well-being of these women.

Services for Black women must meet the needs of the community and be both available and culturally suitable. Effective assessments are crucial. If social workers are not educated about Black women and the best practices with this diverse group, effective and proficient assessment tools may be lacking. Black women will only trust public services if the standards are acceptable to them. Social workers and other clinicians have a responsibility to ensure that social systems are aware of the salience of religion and are responsive to women.

The need to educate the community of the necessity of supporting this segment of the population is imperative. This includes partnering with the faith community, local and national government, and advocating for evidence-based services within the community, such as wellness centers, meditation and yoga practice, and resources for religion-based therapeutic services such as pastoral counseling centers.

This study adds to the growing body of research on religion and Black women. It substantiates comparable studies on the efficacy of religion with Black women. However, it also engenders a comprehension of the nuances of what mental well-being means for Black women, as well as the various interpretations of religion based on the experiences of the women. The study was conducted on a small scale, in a particular geographic area; thus, additional qualitative research on this population would allow scholars to generalize results more easily and locate the mental well-being of Black women within the larger social structure.

The women participated in this study because of their interest in both mental well-being and religion. Further studies are needed to examine the mental well-being of this population without using the construct of religion. This will aid in determining whether religion is a major factor in mental well-being for Black women, and whether the characterizations of religion are comparable. Studies on a larger scale would contribute better comprehension about religion and its connection to mental well-being and allows us to perfect our understanding of cultural differences. In a recent study of 101 Black women, 91% experienced an incident in their lives. Of those who had such an experience, 61%, a majority of the women, qualified it as traumatic. Of this majority, 27% developed posttraumatic stress disorder. A majority (80%) mentioned an avid use of religious resources such as prayer, seeking religious counsel, support of faith community and use of religious teachings.

Several of the women in the current study experienced significant trauma in their lives. Yet they attributed much of their mental well-being to their concept and practice of religion. These women demonstrate great strength and resilience. What might we learn that could transfer to other minority groups?

The demographics of our society are changing. In many urban communities, including Washington, DC, increasing property values are dislocating lower-income families and businesses and replacing them with people with higher income. A Washington, DC, government report revealed that persons with higher income are more likely to remain in the city than lower-income residents. Property values and high rents are displacing low-income persons, and the city and nearby suburbs are becoming a place for the wealthy. Washington, DC is the fastest gentrifying area in the country. Washington, DC is no longer majority Black. The complexion and population of our major urban centers and its suburbs have shifted. Future studies need to incorporate quantitative and qualitative methods to analyze both physical and mental health disparities, economic and social systems, and cultural comprehension. It is then that we will be able to develop human service systems that address more of the factors that contribute to mental well-being.

Researchers need to better understand the protective role of religion and spirituality that can be assessed across different populations while controlling for race as a variable. How is it that people find meaning in their religion? How does religion protect people against sexism and racism?

In providing services for Black women and recognizing the saliency of religion, an understanding of the various ways in which women describe and experience religion can go a long way towards developing interventions to enhance the well-being of these women. Social workers such as clinicians, educators, and developers of social policy can do much to bring improvement to our society.

Black women continue to have an impact in the national and community landscape of our country. It was clear that in the 2020 presidential election that Black women voted and worked to get out the vote to ensure that Joe Biden won the election. Black women continue to be the Democratic Party's most powerful voting group. These are the same women who are concerned about the community as a whole and who work as activists for visible results showing forth their own empowerment. These women use coping mechanisms of faith, religion, and their own deepened spirituality. This demonstrates their resilience and effectiveness in their personal lives and their communities, which impacts our nation. The religious expression of Black women traverses their race, their class, and their gender, which takes them through the traumas of their lives on a journey to wholeness and strength.

Notes

Chapter 1

6: From Delores Carpenter and N. E. Williams, eds., *African American Heritage Hymnal* (Chicago, Illinois: GIA Publications, 2001), 161.

11: Howard University, School of Social Work, "The Black Perspective," https://socialwork.howard.edu/about-us/black-perspective.

11: Donelda Cook and Christine Wiley, "Psychotherapy with Members of African American Churches and Spiritual Traditions," in *Handbook of Psychotherapy and Religious Diversity*, ed. P. Scott Richards and A. E. Bergin (American Psychological Association, 2000), 370.

12: John S. Mbiti, *African Religions and Philosophy* (London, England: Heinemann Educational Publishers, 1969), 108.

12: C. Eric Lincoln and L. H. Mamiya, *The Black Church in the African American Experience* (Duke University Press, 1990).

14: Bettye Collier-Thomas, *Jesus, Jobs, and Justice: African American Women and Religion* (New York, NY: Random House Inc., 2010).

14: Bernice McNair Barnett, "Invisible Southern Black Women Leaders in the Civil Rights Movement: The Triple Constraints of Gender, Race, and Class," *Gender and Society* 7 no. 2 (2016).

14: Rosetta Ross, *Witnessing & Testifying* (Fortress Press, 2003)

18: Valerie Borum, "African American Women's Perceptions of Depression and Suicide and Protection: A Womanist Exploration," *Journal of Women and Social Work* 27, no. 3 (2012).

18: Linda M. Chatters, "Religion and Health: Public Health Research and Practice," *Annual Review of Public Health* 27 (2000).

20: David H Rosmarin, et al., "Attitudes Toward Spirituality/Religion Among Members of the Association for Behavioral and Cognitive Therapies," *Professional Psychology: Research and Practice* 44, no. 6 (2013).

20: R. Schiffman, "More Psychotherapists are Incorporating Religion Into Their Practices," *The Washington Post*, September 23, 2022.

21: D. Wallechinsky, Office of Faith Based Neighborhood Partnerships, https://www.allgov.com.

24: Office of Minority Health (OMH), African American Profile, http://minorityhealth.hhs.gov/templates/browse.aspx-?lvl=2&lvlid=51.

24: Nancy Boyd-Franklin, *Black Families in Therapy*, 2nd ed. (Guilford Press, 2006).

24: Jacqueline S. Mattis, Nyasha A. Grayman-Simpson, "Faith and the Sacred," in *African American Life in APA Handbook of Psychology, Religion and Spirituality: Context Theory and Research*, ed. K. I. Pargament, J. J. Exline, and J. W. Jones (American Psychological Association, 2013), 1.

25: Robert Joseph Taylor, Linda M. Chatters, and Jeff Levin, *Religion in the Lives of African Americans* (Sage, 2004).

25: Theola Labbe-Debose, "Black Women are Among Country's Most Religious Group," *The Washington Post*, July 6, 2012.

Chapter 2

29: Alice Walker, *In Search of our Mothers' Garden: Womanist Prose* (New York: Harcourt, Brace, Jovanovich, Publishers, 1983).

30: Ibid., xi.

30: Monica Coleman, *Making A Way Out of No Way* (Fortress, 2008), 6

31: Layli Phillips, *The Womanist Reader* (Routledge, 2006).

31: Corliss Heath, "A Womanist Approach to Understanding and Assessing the Relationship Between Spirituality and Mental Health," *Mental Health, Religion, and Culture* 9, no. 2 (2006).

31: Rose Marie Hoffman, "Gender Self-Definition and Gender Self-Acceptance in Women: Intersections with Feminist, Womanist, and Ethnic Identities," *Journal of Counseling & Development* 84 (2006).

31: Alice Walker, *In Search of our Mothers' Garden: Womanist Prose* (New York: Harcourt, Brace, Jovanovich, Publishers, 1983), xi.

31: Melanie L. Harris, *Gifts of Virtue, Alice Walker, and Womanist Ethics* (Palgrave Macmillan, 2010).

32: Barbara Bryant Solomon, *Black Empowerment* (Columbia University Press, 1976)

33: Sara Ganim and Linh Tran, "How Tap Water Became Toxic in Flint Michigan," CNN, January 13, 2016, http://www.cnn.com/2016/01/11/health/toxic-tap-water-flint-michigan/.

33: Boyd-Franklin, *Black Families in Therapy.*

34: Barbara Bryant Solomon, *Black Empowerment* (Columbia University Press, 1976).

34: Lorraine M. Gutierrez, "Working with Women of Color: An Empowerment Perspective," *Social Work* 35, no. 2 (1990): 149.

34: Joan Entmacher, et al., *Insecure Unequal: Poverty and Income Among Women and Families 2001–2013* (The National Women's Law Center, 2013).

34 Lorraine Gutierrez, et al., "The Complexity of Community Empowerment," *Journal of Community Practice* 13 no. 2. (2005).

34: Washington Interfaith Network, Jobs Action, February 5, 2013, www.windc-iaf.org.

35: Cheryl Holcomb-McCoy, "Empowerment Groups for Urban African American Girls: A Response," *Professional School Counseling* 8, no. 5. (2005).

Chapter 3

41: The Association of Religion Data Archives, Religious Coping, 2013. https://www.thearda.com/menu-selection-landing-page?topmenu=Research

42: Robert Joseph Taylor, et al., "Nonorganizational Religious Participation, Subjective Religiosity, and Spirituality Among Older African Americans and Black Caribeans," *Journal of Religion and Health* 50 (2011).

42: Peter Hill & Ralph Hood Jr., *Measures of Religiosity* (Birmingham, AL: Religious Education Press, 1999).

42: Kenneth Pargament, et al., "Religious Coping among the Religious: The Relationships Between Religious Coping and Well-being in a National Sample of Presbyterian Clergy, Elders and Members," *Journal of Scientific Study of Religion* 40, no. 3. (2001).

42: Janice Bowie, et al., "The Relationship Between Religious Coping Style and Anxiety Over Breast Cancer in African American Women," *Journal of Religion and Health* 40, no. 4 (2001).

43: Laurence Jackson amd Robert Coursey, "The Relationship of God's Control and Internal Locus of Control to Intrinsic Religious motivation Coping and Purpose in Life," *Journal for the Scientific Study of Religion* 27, no. 3 (1988).

44: Laurie Burke, et al., "Faith in the Wake of Homocide: Religious Coping and Bereavement Distress in an African American Sample," *The International Journal for Psychology of Religion* 21 (2011).

45: Kenneth Pargament, et al., "The Many Methods of Religious Coping: Developmental and Initial Validation of the RCOPE," *Journal of Clinical Psychology* 56 (2000).

Chapter 4

53: Natalie Arnette, et al., "Enhancing Spiritual Well-being Among African American Female Survivors of Intimate Partner Violence," *Journal of Clinical Psychology* 63 (2007).

53: Tricia Bent-Goodley, et al., "A Spirit Unbroken: The Black Church's Evolving Response to Domestic Violence." Social *Work and Christianity* 39 no. 1 (2012).

54: Hilda Davis-Carroll, "An Ethic of Resistance: Choosing Life in Health Messages African American Women," *Journal of Religion and Health* 50 (2011).

55: Ann Fischer & Kenna Bolton Holz, "Testing a Model of Women's Personal Sense of Justice, Control, Well-being, and Distress in the Context of Sexist Discrimination," *Psychology of Women Quarterly* 34 (2010).

56: Carman Williams and Marsha Wiggins, "Womanist Spirituality as a Response to the Racism-Sexism Double Bind in African American Women," *Counseling and Values* 54 (2010).

58: Johnnie Hamilton-Mason, et al., "Some of Us Are Braver: Stress and Coping Among African American Women," *Journal of Human Behavior in the Social Environment* 19 (2009).

59: Olivia Washington, et al., "Five Dimensions of Faith and Spirituality of Older African American Women Transitioning Out of Homelessness," *Journal of Religion and Health* 48 (2009).

64: Washington Interfaith Network, https://www.windc.org/win-issue-agenda-2023/.

65: Besheer Mohamed, et al., "Faith Among Black Americans," Pew Research Center, February 16, 2021, https://www.pewresearch.org/religion/2021/0216/faith-among-black-americans/.

Chapter 5

68: C. Eric Lincoln and Lawrence H. Mamiya, *The Black Church in the African American Experience* (Duke University Press, 1990).

69: Henry Louis Gates, *The Black Church: This Is Our Story, This Is Our Song* (Penguin, 2021).

70: Harold Koenig, et al., eds., *Handbook of Religion and Health*, 2nd ed. (Oxford University Press, 2012).

70: Cook and Wiley, "Psychotherapy with Members of African American Churches and Spiritual Traditions."

70: Donelda Cook, "Psychotherapy and the Power of Religion," in *Handbook of African American Health*, ed. R. L. Hampton, T.P. Gullotta, and R. L. Crowel (Guilford, 2010).

74: Robert Joseph Taylor, et al., *Religion in the Lives of African Americans: Social, Psychological and Health Perspectives* (Sage, 2004).

74: Perry N. Halkitis, et al., "The Meanings and Manifestations of Religion and Spirituality Among Lesbian, Gay, bisexual and Transgender Adults," *Journal of Adult Development* 16 (2009).

75: Peter Hill and Ralph Hood Jr., *Measures of Religiosity* (Religious Education Press, 1999).

75: Natalie Arnette, et al., "Enhancing Spiritual Well-being Among Suicidal African American Female Survivors of Intimate Partner Violence," *Journal of Clinical Psychology* 63 (2007).

75: Craig W. Ellison, "Conceptualization and Measurement," *Journal of Psychology and Theology* 11 (1983).

75: Tricia Bent-Goodley, et al., "A Spirit Unbroken: The Black Church's Evolving Response to Domestic Violence," *Social Work and Christianity* 39, no. 1 (2012).

76: Natalie Arnette, et al., "Enhancing Spiritual Well-being Among Suicidal African American Female Survivors of Intimate Partner Violence," *Journal of Clinical Psychology* 63 (2007).

76: Cook and Wiley, "Psychotherapy with Members of African American Churches and Spiritual Traditions," 370.

79: James A. Davis, et al., "General Social Survey with Cultural, Information Security, and Freedom Modules," National Archive of Data on Arts and Culture, 2002, https://www.icpsr.umich.edu/web/NADAC/studies/35536.

79: Lisa Rappaport, "Meditation May Be Good for Your Heart" *Everyday Health*, 2020.

79: Greg Wilkinson and Mauro Propeizi, "From Sectarian to Holistic: The Practice of Meditation in Modern Japan," *Religion and Spirituality in Modern Society* 5, no. 4 (2015).

80: Emmanuel Oyemomi, "Kyrios in the Fourth Gospel and its Implications for African Asian Ecclesiology," *American Journal of Biblical Theology* 1 (2019).

80: Martin Palmer, *The Jesus Sutras: Rediscovering the lost scrolls of Taoist Christianity* (Ballantine, 2001).

80: Koenig, et al., *Handbook of Religion and Health*.

Chapter 7

97: Mary V. Alfred & Dominique T. Chlup, "Neoliberalism Illiteracy, and Poverty: Framing The Rise in Black Women's Incarceration" The Western Journal of Black Studies 33 no. 4 (2009).

97: Barbara Bryant Solomon, *Black Empowerment* (Columbia University Press, 1976).

98: Zora N. Hurston, *Their Eyes Were Watching God* (Virago, 2018).

Chapter 8

107: Monique Moultrie, *Passionate and Pious: Religious Media and Black Women's Sexuality* (Duke University Press, 2017).

107: "Mammy, Jezebel, and Sapphire: Stereotyping Black Women in Media," *Al Jazeera*, July 26, 2020, https://www.aljazeera.com/program/the-listening-post/2020/7/26/mammy-jezebel-and-sapphire-stereotyping-black-women-in-media.

108: Ibid.

108: Cheryl Woods-Giscombe, "Superwoman Schema: African American Women's Views on Stress, Strength, and Health," *Qualitative Health Research* 20 no. 5 (2010).

110: Sara Matsuzaka, et al., "Black Women's Social Media Use, Integration and Social Media Addiction," *Social Media + Society* 9, no. 1 (2023).

110: Jadesola Olayinka, et al., "#BlackGirlMagic: Impact of the Social Media Movement on Black Women's Self-esteem," *International Journal of Women's Dermatology* 7, no. 2 (2021).

111: Taylor, et al. "Nonorganizational Religious Participation."

112: Jacqueline Salmon, "Rift Over Gay Unions Reflects Battle New to Black Churches," *The Washington Post*, August 8, 2019.

112: Christine and Dennis Wiley, "Gay Marriage In our Black Church," *The Washington Post*, January 2, 2010.

113: Ashton Crawley, "The Future of the Black Church and Its Ability to Reckon With Its Gay Members," *The Washington Post*, August 20, 2021.

Chapter 9

116: Kiana Cox and Jeff Diamant, "Black Men are Less Religious Than Black Women, But More Religious Than White Women and Men," Pew Research Center, September 26, 2018.

116: Nyasha Grayman-Simpson and Jacqueline Mattis, "If It Wasn't For the Church...: Organizational Religiosity and Informal Community Helping Among African American Adults," *Journal of African American Studies* 17 no. 3 (2012).

116: Linda Chatters, "Religion and Health: Public Health Research and Practice," *Annual Review of Public Health* 21 (2000).

116: "Theories Explaining Gender Differences in Religion," Pew Research Center, March 22, 2016, https://www.pewresearch.org/religion/2016/03/22/theories-explaining-gender-differences-in-religion/.

117: Taylor, et al., *Religion in the Lives of African Americans.*

117: Wendy Sawyer and Peter Wagner, "Mass Incarceration: The Whole Pie 2024," Prison Policy Initiative, March 14, 2024, https://www.prisonpolicy.org/reports/pie2024.html

Chapter 10

121: Jesse Washington, "Blacks Struggle with 72% Unwed Mothers Rate," Associated Press, November 7, 2010, https://www.nbcnews.com/id/wbna39993685.

122: Edna Brown, et al., "Religiosity as a Moderator of Family Conflict and Depressive Symptoms Among African American and White Young Grandmothers," *Journal of Human Behavior in the Social Environment* 14, no. 4 (2008).

123: Patricia Hill Collins, "The Meaning of Motherhood in Black Culture and Black Mother/ Daughter Relationships," in *Toward a New Psychology of Gender: A Reader*, ed. Mary M. Gergen and Sara N. Davis (Routledge 1997).

123: Ibid., 325.

123: Sandra Edmonds Crewe and Anita Stowell Ritter, "Grandparents Raising Grandchildren in the District of Columbia: Focus Group Report," AARP, 2003.

124: Besheer Mohammed, et al., "Faith Among Black Americans," Pew Research Center, February 16, 2021, https://www.pewresearch.org/religion/wp-content/uploads/sites/7/2021/02/PF_02.16.21_Black.religion.report.pdf.

126: Dani McClain, *We Live for the We: The Political Power of Black Motherhood* (Bold Type Books, 2019), 179.

Chapter 11

129: Jacqueline Grant, *White Women's Christ and Black Women's Jesus: Feminist Christology and Womanist Response* (Scholars Press, 1989).

129: Yolanda Pierce, *In My Grandmother's House: Black Women, Faith, and the Stories We Inherit* (Broadleaf Books, 2023), 51.

Chapter 12

137: Malcolm Gladwell, *David and Goliath* (Back Bay Books, 2013).

138: "Modeling the Future of Religion in America," Pew Research Center, September 13, 2022, https://www.pewresearch.org/religion/2022/09/13/modeling-the-future-of-religion-in-america/.

139: Council on Social Work Education, Religion and Spirituality Clearinghouse, 2013.

139: Dorothy Graff, "A Study of Baccalaureate Social Work Students' Beliefs About the Inclusion Of Religious and Spiritual Content in Social Work," *Journal of Social Work Education* 43, no. 2 (2007).

140: Heyman, et al., "Social Workers' Attitudes toward the Role of Religion and Spirituality in Social Work Practice," *Journal of Pastoral Care & Counseling* 41 (2006).

140: Council on Social Work Education, "Engage Diversity and Difference in Practice," 2015, https://www.cswe.org/getmedia/23a35a39-78c7-453f-b805-b67f1dca2ee5/2015-epas-and-glossary.pdf.

141: Koenig, et al., *Handbook of Religion and Health.*

141: Cook and Christine Wiley, "Psychotherapy with Members of African American Churches and Spiritual Traditions."

141: Valerie Borum, "African American Women's Perceptions of Depression and Suicide and Protection: A Womanist Exploration," *Journal of Women and Social Work* 27, no. 3 (2012).

142: Regina G. Davis, et al., "Treatment Barriers for Low-income, Urban African Americans with Undiagnosed Posttraumatic Stress Disorder," *Journal of Traumatic Stress* 21, no. 2 (2008).

142: K. B. Wogan, "Low-income Residents More Likely to Leave DC," 2015, https://www.governing.com/archive/gov-low-income-residents-district-columbia.html.